Tissue Plasminogen Activator in Thrombolytic Therapy

Tissue Plasminogen Activator in Thrombolytic Therapy

edited by

Burton E. Sobel
Washington University School of Medicine
St. Louis, Missouri

Désiré Collen
University of Leuven
Leuven, Belgium
and University of Vermont College of Medicine
Burlington, Vermont

Elliott B. Grossbard
Genentech, Inc.
South San Francisco, California

MARCEL DEKKER, INC.   New York and Basel

Library of Congress Cataloging-in-Publication Data

Tissue plasminogen activator in thrombolytic therapy.

Includes bibliographies and index.
1. Thrombosis--Chemotherapy. 2. Tissue
plasminogen activator--Therapeutic use. I. Sobel,
Burton E. II. Collen, D. (Désiré) III. Grossbard,
Elliott B. [DNLM: 1. Plasminogen
Activator, Tissue-Type--therapeutic use. 2. Thrombosis--
drug therapy. WH 310 T616]
RC694.3.T57 1987   616.1'35061   87-501
ISBN 0-8247-7666-6

Marcel Dekker, Inc.
270 Madison Avenue, New York, New York 10016

Current printing (last digit):
10 9 8 7 6 5 4 3 2 1

PRINTED IN THE UNITED STATES OF AMERICA

Preface

The field of thrombolysis has evoked intense interest over the past 3 years, prompted in large part by studies with recombinant tissue plasminogen activator (rt-PA). Since the first patient was treated in February 1984, more than 3000 patients have been treated in the United States, Europe, Australia, Canada, New Zealand, and Japan.

Since the clinical literature on rt-PA is dispersed through many journals covering different clinical disciplines, and since such literature often lags behind clinical developments, we have tried in this volume to collect the clinical experience of investigators in the thrombolysis field who have worked with or supervised trials utilizing rt-PA in a variety of clinical indications.

The book proceeds through a review of the biology, clinical pharmacology, and pharmacokinetics of tissue plasminogen activator with special attention to rt-PA, followed by a review of the clinical experience accumulated over the last 2½ years in myocardial infarction, pulmonary embolism, venous thrombosis, and peripheral arterial occlusion.

We hope that cardiologists, internists, vascular specialists, and radiologists will find the clinical results described herein of practical value as well as of interest.

We would like to acknowledge the invaluable contribution of the scientists at Genentech whose accomplishments in the fields of molecular biology, protein chemistry, and process sciences are evident in the amazingly rapid progress of rt-PA from an idea to a pharmaceutical.

Finally, we are grateful to the authors for their clinical skills, their participation in the research, and their contributions to this book.

Burton E. Sobel
Désiré Collen
Elliott B. Grossbard

Introduction

The fibrinolytic activity associated with tissue-type plasminogen activator (t-PA) was identified in the 1940s, but significant advances in the understanding of its mechanism of action and therapeutic application of this natural product required breakthroughs in protein chemistry and molecular biology that did not occur until several decades later.

In 1980 Rijken was able to develop a procedure that yielded 1 mg of t-PA from 5 kg of human uterine tissue (1). Utilizing a modification of this procedure, Rijken and Collen were able to purify gram quantities of t-PA from a melanoma cell line. Although extraordinarily labor-intensive, these procedures produced sufficient quantities of highly purified t-PA for extensive biological, biochemical, and physiological studies of the material (2). During the course of these studies, the stimulation of t-PA activity by and high affinity of t-PA for fibrin were elucidated and mechanisms accounting for the relative clot specificity of t-PA were formulated (3).

In 1981 Weimar and Collen reported two patients with renal vein thrombosis who were treated successfully with low doses of t-PA (5 and 7.5 mg over 24 hr) (4). As often occurs, subsequent courses of therapy in succeeding patients were less successful, but the initial report stimulated interest in the potential of t-PA as a pharmaceutical.

Scientists from Genentech learned of Collen's work and a collaboration ensued that resulted in the successful cloning and expression of the human t-PA gene (5). The product was called recombinant human tissue-type plasminogen activator (rt-PA).

Scientists at Genentech discovered that a mammalian tissue culture system (Chinese hamster ovary cells) was the best biological factory for the expression of the human t-PA gene, and when rt-PA was studied in canine and primate coronary thrombosis models, the results confirmed similar studies conducted with melanoma-derived t-PA (6–9).

In 1983, seven patients with acute myocardial infarction were treated with melanoma-derived t-PA, and six exhibited prompt coronary thrombolysis (10). The results from this study, along with those from studies in dogs and primates, provided a foundation for investigators from the Johns Hopkins Medical Institutions, Massachusetts General Hospital, Washington University, and Genentech to formulate a protocol for a multicenter trial initiated in February 1984 (11). The rt-PA used in this trial was produced with a technology appropriate for clinical trials, but not of sufficient scale for commercialization. This rt-PA, given the code number G11021, was predominantly in the two-chain form, i.e., two polypeptide chains held together by a single disulfide bond.

In June of 1984, the National Heart, Lung and Blood Institute (NHLBI) commenced a pilot trial with rt-PA (G11021), which confirmed the results of the Genentech-sponsored trial (12). The NHLBI study group [Thrombolysis in Myocardial Infarction (TIMI)] then proceeded to conduct a prospective randomized double-blind trial comparing rt-PA to streptokinase. The trial was stopped before completion on the recommendation of the NHLBI Policy Board because of the obvious superiority of rt-PA (13).

By March 1985, Phase I of the TIMI trial was over and Genentech had scaled up its process for the manufacture of rt-PA. The rt-PA produced by this commercial process (G11035, G11044) was predominantly single-chain (60–80%) and had a shorter half-life than G11021, two facts that appear *not* to be causally related (Baughman R, Hotchkiss A, personal communication). Pharmacokinetic considerations led to a dosage change in subsequent phases of the TIMI trial (14). The finding was concurrently confirmed by Garabedian and co-workers (15).

Elliott B. Grossbard, M.D.
Director, Clinical Research
Genentech, Inc.
South San Francisco, California

REFERENCES

1. Rijken DC, Wijngaards G, Zaal-Dejong M, et al: Biochem Biophys Acta 580: 140, 1979.
2. Collen D, Rijken DC, Van Damme J, et al: Thromb Haemost 48:294, 1982.
3. Hoylaerts M, Rijken DC, Lijnen HR, et al: J Biol Chem 257:2912, 1982.
4. Weimar W, Stibbe J, van Seyen AJ, et al: Lancet 2:1018, 1981.
5. Pennica D, Holmes WE, Kohr WJ, et al: Nature 201:214, 1983.
6. Bergmann SR, Fox KAA, Ter-Pogossian, et al: Science 220:1181, 1983.
7. Van de Werf F, Bergmann JR, Fox KAA, et al: Circulation 69:605, 1984.
8. Gold HK, Fallon JT, Yasuda T, et al: Circulation 70:700, 1984.
9. Flameng W, Van de Werf F, Vanhaecke J, et al: J Clin Invest 75:84, 1985.
10. Van de Werf F, Ludbrook PA, Bergmann SR, et al: N Engl J Med 310:609, 1984.
11. Collen D, Topol EJ, Tiefenbrunn AJ, et al: Circulation 70:1012, 1984.
12. Williams DO, Borer J, Braunwald EB, et al: Circulation 73:338, 1986.
13. The TIMI Study Group: N Engl J Med 312:932, 1985.
14. Mueller H for the TIMI Study: Clin Res 34:631A, 1986.
15. Garabedian H, Gold HK, Leinbach RC, et al: J Am Coll Cardiol, in press.

Contents

MYOCARDIAL INFARCTION

VENOUS THROMBOEMBOLISM AND PERIPHERAL VASCULAR OCCLUSION

THE EUROPEAN AND JAPANESE EXPERIENCE

Contributors

Robert A. Baughman, Jr., Pharm.D., Ph.D. Scientist, Department of Pharmacological Sciences, Genentech, Inc., South San Francisco, California

Eugene Braunwald, M.D., M.A.(Hon.), M.D.(Hon.) Hersey Professor of the Theory and Practice of Physic and Herman Ludwig Blumgart Professor of Medicine, Harvard Medical School, and Chairman, Department of Medicine, Brigham and Women's Hospital, Boston, Massachusetts

Désiré Collen, M.D., Ph.D. Professor of Medicine, Department of Medical Research, Center for Thrombosis and Vascular Research, University of Leuven, Leuven, Belgium, and Professor of Biochemistry and Medicine, University of Vermont College of Medicine, Burlington, Vermont

William Ganz, M.D., C.Sc. Professor, Department of Medicine, University of California at Los Angeles School of Medicine, and Senior Scientist, Division of Cardiology, Cedars-Sinai Medical Center, Los Angeles, California

Herman K. Gold, M.D.   Associate Physician and Co-Director of Cardiac Catheterization Laboratory, Cardiac Unit, Department of Medicine, Massachusetts General Hospital, and Associate Professor, Department of Medicine, Harvard Medical School, Boston, Massachusetts

Samuel Z. Goldhaber, M.D.   Assistant Professor, Department of Medicine, Harvard Medical School, and Associate Physician, Brigham and Women's Hospital, Boston, Massachusetts

Robert A. Graor, M.D.   Staff, Department of Peripheral Vascular Medicine, Cleveland Clinic, Cleveland, Ohio

Hirofumi Kambara, M.D.   Associate Professor, Third Division, Department of Internal Medicine, Faculty of Medicine, Kyoto University, Kyoto, Japan

Chuichi Kawai, M.D.   Professor and Director, Third Division, Department of Internal Medicine, Faculty of Medicine, Kyoto University, Kyoto, Japan

Robert C. Leinbach, M.D.   Associate Professor, Department of Medicine, Massachusetts General Hospital and Harvard Medical School, Boston, Massachusetts

William W. O'Neill, M.D.   Assistant Professor, Department of Internal Medicine, and Director, Cardiac Catheterization Laboratory, University of Michigan Medical School, Ann Arbor, Michigan

Eugene R. Passamani, M.D.   Associate Director for Cardiology, Division of Heart and Vascular Diseases, National Heart, Lung and Blood Institute, Bethesda, Maryland

Barbara Risius, M.D.   Staff, Department of Diagnostic Radiology, Cleveland Clinic, Cleveland, Ohio

Burton E. Sobel, M.D.   Lewin Professor of Medicine and Director, Cardiovascular Division, Washington University School of Medicine, St. Louis, Missouri

H. J. C. Swan, M.D., Ph.D.   Director, Division of Cardiology, Department of Medicine, Cedars-Sinai Medical Center, Los Angeles, California

Alan J. Tiefenbrunn, M.D. Associate Professor of Medicine, Cardiovascular Division, Washington University School of Medicine, St. Louis, Missouri

Eric J. Topol, M.D., F.A.C.P., F.A.C.C. Co-Director, Interventional Cardiology, and Assistant Professor, Division of Cardiology, Department of Internal Medicine, University of Michigan Medical School, Ann Arbor, Michigan

Alexander G. G. Turpie, M.D., F.A.C.P., F.R.C.P.C. Professor, Department of Medicine, McMaster University and Hamilton General Hospital, Hamilton, Ontario, Canada

Marc Verstraete, M.D., Ph.D. Doctor, Department of Medical Research, Center for Thrombosis and Vascular Research, University of Leuven, Leuven, Belgium

PHARMACOLOGY

1

Biological Properties of Plasminogen Activators

Désiré Collen
University of Leuven
Leuven, Belgium
and University of Vermont College of Medicine
Burlington, Vermont

I. MAIN COMPONENTS OF THE FIBRINOLYTIC SYSTEM

The fibrinolytic system, schematically represented in Figure 1, contains a proenzyme, plasminogen, which can be converted to the active enzyme plasmin by several different types of plasminogen activators. Inhibition of the fibrinolytic system can occur at the level of either the plasminogen activators or plasmin. The definition and nomenclature of these components are summarized in Table 1.

Plasminogen

Physicochemical Properties

Human plasminogen is a single-chain glycoprotein consisting of 790 amino acids. It contains 24 disulfide bridges and five homologous triple-loop structures, or "kringles" (1). Native plasminogen has amino-terminal glutamic acid ("Glu-plasminogen") but is easily converted by limited plasmic digestion to modified forms, commonly designated "Lys-plasminogen," by hydrolysis of the Arg 67-Met 68, Lys 76-Lys 77, or Lys 77-Val 78 peptide bonds.

3

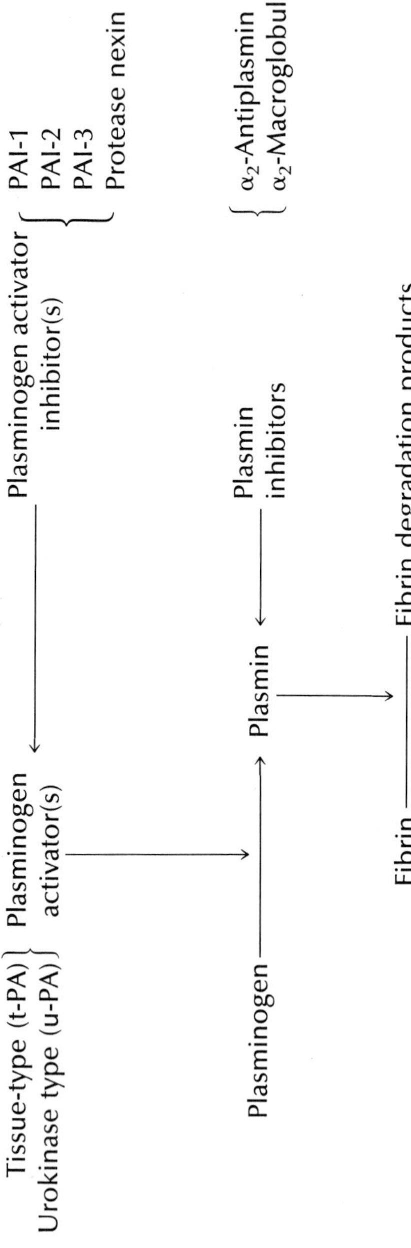

Figure 1 Schematic representation of the fibrinolytic system.

Table 1   Components of the Fibrinolytic System

Plasminogen	Proenzyme form of the fibrinolytic enzyme
Plasmin	Active fibrinolytic enzyme
Streptokinase	Streptococcal protein that activates the fibrinolytic system in human plasma indirectly
Urokinase	Plasminogen activator isolated from urine or kidney cell cultures, consisting of two polypeptide chains; different from tissue-type plasminogen activator
Tissue-type plasminogen activator (t-PA)	Enzyme present in tissues that converts plasminogen to plasmin; identical or similar to blood plasminogen activator and vascular plasminogen activator
Single-chain urokinase-type plasminogen activator (scu-PA)	Enzyme present in blood and urine, related to urokinase but consisting of a single-chain M_r 54,000 polypeptide
α_2-Antiplasmin	Specific fast-reacting plasmin inhibitor in human plasma
Plasminogen activator inhibitor-1	Fast-acting inhibitor of tissue-type plasminogen activator (and urokinase) in blood and secreted by endothelial cells
Plasminogen activator inhibitor-2	Fast acting inhibitor of urokinase and t-PA isolated from placenta and present in blood in late pregnancy
Plasminogen activator inhibitor-3	Inhibitor of urokinase and thrombin, present in plasma and urine, stimulated by heparin

The concentration of plasminogen in plasma is about 2 μM (2). Plasminogen can be assayed in plasma following activation with streptokinase and measurement of the plasminogen-streptokinase complex with a chromogenic substrate (3) or with immunological methods. The method of choice for the purification of human plasminogen is by affinity chromatography on insolubilized lysine, a method introduced by Deutsch and Mertz (4).

Activation to Plasmin

Conversion of Plasminogen to Plasmin.   Lys-plasminogen forms are converted to plasmin by cleavage of a single Arg-Val bond (5) corresponding to the Arg 560-Val 561 bond. The two-chain plasmin molecule is composed of a heavy chain, or A-chain, originating from the amino-terminal part of plasminogen, and a light chain, or B-chain, constituting the carboxy-terminal part (6). The B-chain contains an active site similar to that of trypsin, which is composed of His 602, Asp 645, and Ser 740 (1).

Activation of Glu-plasminogen to plasmin by urokinase in purified systems occurs about 20 times slower than activation of Lys-plasminogen, but in either case Lys-plasmin is formed. Wiman and Wallen (7) initially proposed that activation of Glu-plasminogen occurs in two steps: release of the amino-terminal ''preactivation'' peptide mainly by cleavage at Arg 67-Met 68, yielding Lys-plasminogen, followed by cleavage of the Arg 560-Val 561 bond to generate plasmin. Holvoet et al. (8), however, recently provided evidence that activation of plasminogen to plasmin in vivo occurs by hydrolysis of the Arg 560-Val 561 bond in Glu-plasminogen and not via formation of the Lys-plasminogen intermediate.

Activation with Urokinase and Streptokinase. The activation of human plasminogen by urokinase or by the streptokinase-plasminogen complex obeys Michaelis-Menten kinetics. Both for streptokinase and urokinase, kinetic parameters have been reported ranging over at least two orders of magnitude for K_M and one order of magnitude for k_{cat}. In one study (9), activation of plasminogen with the Glu-plasminogen-streptokinase complex occurs with a K_M of 0.12 μM and k_{cat} of 0.15 s^{-1}, as compared with values of 1.4 μM for K_M and 0.7 s^{-1} for k_{cat} for the activation with urokinase (9). Activation of Lys-plasminogen by streptokinase (9) or urokinase (10) appears to be three to 10 times faster than that of Glu-plasminogen. In the presence of certain omega-aminocarboxylic acids, e.g., 6-aminohexanoic acid, the rate of activation of Glu-plasminogen by urokinase increases 10- to 20-fold, whereas that of Lys-plasminogen is unaffected.

Activation with Tissue-Type Plasminogen Activator. The activation of plasminogen by tissue-type plasminogen activator obeys Michaelis-Menten kinetics with more favorable kinetic constants in the presence of fibrin than in its absence (11,12). Hoylaerts et al. (11) found a marked decrease of K_M in the presence of fibrin (from 65 to 0.16 μM), while the catalytic rate constant did not change significantly (k_{cat} from 0.06 to 0.1 s^{-1}). Similar results were obtained using CNBr-digested fibrinogen as a stimulator (13). Ranby (12) reported a change in K_M (from 7.6 to 0.18 μM) as well as in k_{cat} (from 0.008 to 0.12 s^{-1}); also, Nieuwenhuizen et al. (14) found that both k_{cat} (from 0.002 to 0.058 s^{-1}) and K_M (from 0.053 to 0.003 μM) change on addition of fibrin to the incubation mixture.

On initial fibrin degradation, a strong plasminogen binding site is disclosed, resulting in an increased rate of plasmin formation (15). This is supported by the observation of a decrease in K_M from 2 to 0.2 μM during the fibrinolytic process (16).

Tissue-type plasminogen activator (t-PA) occurs as a single-chain molecule or as a proteolytically degraded two-chain form. Although the single-chain form is less active toward low-molecular-weight substrates and inhibitors, the two forms are equally active toward plasminogen (17). The single-chain t-PA is quickly converted to a two-chain form on the fibrin surface (17). This suggests that physiological fibrinolysis induced by native one-chain t-PA occurs mainly via the two-chain derivative, but this conversion does not seem to play a role in the regulation of fibrinolysis.

Activation with Single-Chain Urokinase-Type Plasminogen Activator.   Single-chain urokinase-type plasminogen activator (scu-PA) has a very low activity toward low M_r substrates for urokinase although in mixtures of scu-PA and plasminogen, both urokinase and plasmin are readily generated (18–20).

A kinetic analysis of the activation of plasminogen by scu-PA (20) has revealed that it can be represented by three sequential reactions that all obey Michaelis-Menten kinetics: 1) direct activation of plasminogen by scu-PA, with K_M = 0.03 μM and k_{cat} = 0.02 s^{-1}, 2) activation of scu-PA by generated plasmin with K_M = 3.3 μM and k_{cat} = 1.4 s^{-1}, and 3) activation of plasminogen by generated urokinase with K_M = 25 μM and k_{cat} = 1.0 s^{-1}. In this model, scu-PA formally behaves as an enzyme in the first reaction, with a high affinity for its substrate plasminogen but with a low catalytic rate constant. The high stability of the scu-PA plasminogen complex (low K_M) is exceptional among serine proteases.

Lysine Binding Sites

The plasminogen molecule contains structures called lysine binding sites, which interact specifically with certain amino acids such as lysine, 6-aminohexanoic acid, and trans-4-amino-methylcyclohexane-1-carboxylic acid (tranexamic acid) (21,22). These lysine binding sites are located in the plasmin A-chain (23). The high-affinity lysine binding site is contained within the first three kringle structures of plasminogen (24)—most probably in the first kringle.

Plasminogen can specifically bind to fibrin through its lysine binding sites. Both in purified systems (25) and in plasma (26), Lys-plasminogen has a higher affinity for fibrin than for Glu-plasminogen. The presence of 6-aminohexanoic acid abolishes the adsorption of plasminogen to fibrin.

The lysine binding sites of plasmin(ogen) also mediate its interaction with α_2-antiplasmin and with histidine-rich glycoprotein. On the basis of these interactions, it was suggested that the lysine binding sites play a crucial role in the regulation of fibrinolysis (27).

Plasminogen Activators

Plasminogen activators are serine proteases with a high specificity for plasminogen. They hydrolyze the Arg 560-Val 561 peptide bond in the inactive proenzyme plasminogen, yielding the active two-chain serine protease plasmin. Several pathways of plasminogen activation have been identified. Some of these activators are counteracted by inhibitors.

"Intrinsic" Activation

In the intrinsic or humoral pathway of plasminogen activation, all the components involved (factor XII, prekallikrein, high-molecular-weight kininogen) are present in precursor forms in the blood. Several inhibitors of "intrinsic" plasminogen activation occur in human plasma: C_1-inactivator, an inhibitor of factor XIIa-induced fibrinolysis, heparin-antithrombin III complex, and α_2-macroglobulin. The present knowledge of the pathways of "intrinsic" plasminogen activation, which is still incomplete, has been reviewed (28). Its biological role, however, has not been established.

Urokinase

Urokinase-type plasminogen activator (u-PA) is a trypsin-like serine protease composed of two polypeptide chains (M_r 20,000 and 34,000) connected by a single disulfide bridge. It is isolated from human urine or cultured human embryonic kidney cells. Urokinase activates plasminogen directly to plasmin. It may occur in two molecular forms designated S_1 (M_r 31,600, low-molecular-weight urokinase) and S_2 (M_r 54,000, high-molecular-weight urokinase), the former being a proteolytic degradation product of the latter (29). The complete primary structure of high-molecular-weight urokinase has been elucidated (30,31). The light chain contains 157 amino acids (158, including the carboxy-terminal lysine) and the heavy chain 253.

The gene of human urokinase was recently cloned and expressed in *Escherichia coli* (32,33). The complete 2304-base pair cDNA sequence of the gene coding for urokinase contains an open reading frame, beginning with the ATG codon at nucleotides 77 to 79, which extends for 1293 nucleotides until a TGA stop codon is reached at positions 1370 to 1372. The open reading frame is preceded by at least 76 nucleotides of 5' untranslated mRNA and followed by 932 nucleotides of 3' untranslated mRNA. The mRNA codes for a protein of 431 amino acids, of which the first 20 amino acids preceding the mature form of u-PA constitute a typical eukaryotic hydrophobic signal peptide.

The urokinase molecule contains three domains. The first is a cysteine-rich amino-terminal region (residues 5 to 49), which is homologous with epidermal growth factor and which also occurs in t-PA (residues 44 to 91), bovine factor X (54–88), bovine factor IX (2–49), bovine protein C (52–96), and murine and human epidermal growth factor (2–49). The second is a kringle region comprising amino acid residues 50–136, which also occurs five times in plasminogen and twice in prothrombin and in t-PA. The third is a serine protease part with the active site residues His, Asp, and Ser in positions 204, 255, and 356, respectively, which constitutes the carboxy-terminal region of the molecule. Generation of two-chain urokinase occurs by hydrolysis of the Lys 158-Ile 159 peptide bond. Although it was initially assumed that this conversion was a prerequisite for biological function (32), it was subsequently shown that the single-chain form of urokinase has intrinsic fibrin-specific plasminogen activating properties (19,20).

Urokinase has successfully been used for thrombolytic therapy, but its exact place in the management of thrombosis remains to be further established (34).

Streptokinase

Streptokinase is a nonenzyme protein with M_r 47,000 produced by Lancefield group C strains of beta-hemolytic streptococci, which activates the fibrinolytic system indirectly (35). Streptokinase initially forms a 1:1 stoichiometric complex with plasminogen which then undergoes a transition, and exposes an active site in the modified plasminogen moiety, whereby the complex becomes a potent plasminogen activator (36,37).

Streptokinase is at present the most widely used thrombolytic agent, because it is easier to obtain and far less expensive than urokinase. Although streptokinase has been used for thrombolysis for 30 years, its optimal dose regimen and exact place in the treatment of thromboembolic disease are still debated (34).

Tissue-Type Plasminogen Activator

Physicochemical Properties. Native t-Pa is a serine protease composed of one polypeptide chain containing 527 amino acids (38). On limited plasmic action, the molecule is converted to a two-chain activator linked by one disulfide bond (39). This occurs by cleavage of the Arg 275-Ile 176 peptide bond yielding a heavy chain (M_r 31,000) derived from the amino-terminal part of the molecule and a light chain (M_r 28,000) comprising the carboxy-terminal region.

The catalytic site located in the light chain of t-PA is composed of His 322, Asp 371, and Ser 478. The amino acid sequences surrounding these residues are highly homologous to corresponding parts of other serine proteases such as trypsin, thrombin, plasmin, and elastase. The primary structures of high-molecular-weight urokinase and t-PA have a high degree of homology, except that t-PA contains a 43-residue-long amino-terminal region, which has no counterpart in urokinase; this segment is homologous with the finger domains responsible for the fibrin affinity of fibronectin. Limited proteolysis of this region leads to a loss of the fibrin affinity of the enzyme (40). The sequence representing residues 44 to 91 of t-PA is homologous with high-molecular-weight urokinase (residues 5 to 49), bovine factor X (residues 54 to 88), bovine factor IX (residues 54 to 87), bovine protein C (residues 52 to 96), murine epidermal growth factor (residues 2 to 49), and human epidermal growth factor (residues 2 to 49). The heavy chain contains two regions of 82 amino acids each (residues 92 to 173 and 180 to 261) that share a high degree of homology with the five kringles of plasminogen and with similar kringles in prothrombin and urokinase.

The complete 2530-base pair cDNA sequence of t-PA contains a single open reading frame, beginning with the ATG codon at nucleotides 85 to 87, which is followed, 562 codons later, by a TGA termination triplet at nucleotides 1771 to 1773. The serine residue designated as the amino-terminal amino acid is preceded by 35 amino acids, 20 to 23 of which probably constitute a hydrophobic signal peptide. The remaining 12 to 15 hydrophobic amino acids immediately preceding the start of mature t-PA may constitute a ''pro'' sequence similar to that found for serum albumin. The 3' untranslated region of 759 nucleotides contains an AATAAA (positions 2496 to 2501) polyadenylation signal (38).

Ny et al. (41) have shown that the human t-PA gene is split into at least 14 exons by at least 13 introns. Nine introns separate the nonprotease amino-terminal part of the molecule into structural domains. The exon-intron pattern of the B-chain is similar to that of other serine proteases such as trypsin, chymotrypsin, and elastase.

The one- and two-chain forms of t-PA have different amidolytic activities toward low-molecular-weight substrates (42). They have, however, virtually the same fibrinolytic activity (clot lysis) in a purified system and plasminogen-activating properties (17). It has been speculated that the enzymatic activity of the one-chain form may arise from the presence of an epsilon-amino group in the side chain of the lysine residue in the second position of the B-chain (38), which may substitute for the α-amino group generated by conversion of the one-chain precursor molecules to the two-chain serine proteases.

Release and Inhibition.   The concept that t-PA in blood originates from vascular endothelial cells is supported by the finding that endothelial cells in culture secrete plasminogen activator (43), which may, however, be either t-PA or urokinase-like (44). Plasminogen activator, which is enhanced after physical exercise and venous occlusion, is immunologically related to t-PA (45).

t-PA is resistant to the protease inhibitors aprotinin and soybean trypsin inhibitor, which do not react with either the single-or the two-chain form. The protease inhibitors α_2-antiplasmin, C_1-esterase inhibitor, α_1-antitrypsin, and α_2-macroglobulin react slowly with t-PA but these reactions do not appear to be of physiological importance. Inhibitory substances that rapidly react with t-PA have recently been discovered in endothelial cell cultures (46), placental tissue (47), and blood plasma (48–50).

The mechanisms involved in the removal of t-PA from the blood are multiple and poorly understood. One main mechanism of removal of t-PA from the blood is through clearance by the liver, which results in a $t_{1/2}$ of a few minutes (51).

Mechanism of Action.   t-PA is a trypsin-like serine protease, which hydrolyses several tripeptide substrates with arginine as the COOH-terminal amino acid. When t-PA is present during formation of fibrin clots of increasing density, half-maximal binding occurs at approximately 0.14 g fibrin per L (0.4 μM) (17). Kinetic experiments on plasminogen activation in the presence of varying amounts of fibrin suggested a dissociation constant of 0.14 μM (11). Detailed binding studies are, however, still lacking, as is the localization of the binding sites, both in the fibrin molecule and in t-PA.

t-PA is a poor enzyme in the absence of fibrin, but fibrin strikingly enhances the activation rate of plasminogen. This has been explained by an increased affinity of fibrin-bound t-PA for plasminogen without significant influence on the catalytic efficiency of the enzyme (11). The kinetic data of Hoylaerts et al. (11) support a mechanism in which t-PA and plasminogen adsorb to a fibrin clot in a sequential and ordered way, yielding a ternary complex. Fibrin essentially increases the local plasminogen concentration by creating an additional interation between t-PA and its substrate. The high affinity of t-PA for plasminogen in the presence of fibrin thus allows efficient activation on the fibrin clot, while no efficient plasminogen activation by t-PA occurs in plasma.

t-PA occurs either as a single-chain molecule or as a proteolytically degraded two-chain molecule. In contrast to analogous enzyme systems, single-chain t-PA is not, however, an inactive precursor but an active enzyme. Although the single-chain form is less active toward low-molecular-weight substrates and inhibitors, the two forms are almost equally active toward plasminogen (12,17).

Functional domains responsible for the fibrin-binding and catalytic activity of t-PA have been localized in the t-PA molecule. Holvoet et al. partially reduced two-chain t-PA and separated the A- and B-chain (52). The purified B-chain activated plasminogen following Michaelis-Menten kinetics with kinetic constants similar to those of intact t-PA, but fibrin did not stimulate the activation of plasminogen by the B-chain. The purified A-chain bound to fibrin with an affinity similar to that of intact t-PA but did not activate plasminogen.

Single-Chain Urokinase-Type Plasminogen Activator

Bernik (53) had already suggested in 1973 that urokinase might be secreted in an inactive form that can be activated by plasmin, and subsequently Nolan et al. (54) reported that urokinase was secreted by human embryonic kidney cells in a precursor form. More recently, several groups have isolated a single-chain form or urokinase from urine (55,56), plasma (57), and conditioned cell culture media (58–61).

Physicochemical Properties.   scu-PA is a single-chain glycoprotein containing 411 amino acids with 24 cysteine residues (31,33). Hydrolysis of the Lys 158-Ile 159 peptide bond by plasmin converts the molecule to urokinase, a two-chain molecule linked by one disulfide bridge. The catalytic center is located in the carboxy-terminal chain and is composed of Asp 255, His 204, and Ser 356. The amino-terminal chain contains a region homologous to human epidermal growth factor (residues 5–49) and one region homologous to the plasminogen kringles. A low M_r two-chain urokinase (M_r 33,000) can be generated by hydrolysis of the Lys 135-Lys 136 peptide bond following previous cleavage of the Lys 158-Ile 159 bond. A M_r 32,000 form of scu-PA can be generated by specific hydrolysis of the Glu 143-Leu 144 peptide bond in scu-PA by an unidentified protease (62).

scu-PA has a very low reactivity toward low-molecular-weight synthetic substrates or active-site titrants that are very reactive toward urokinase (55–58).

A cDNA for human urokinase was recently cloned and expressed in *E. coli* (32,33). The purified translation product normally consists of active two-chain urokinase, but a single-chain form may be obtained if proteolytic degradation is carefully avoided during purification.

Mechanism of Action.   In mixtures of scu-PA and plasminogen, both urokinase and plasmin are quickly generated. Addition of plasmin inhibitors abolishes the conversion of scu-PA to urokinase but not the activation of plasminogen to plasmin, suggesting that scu-PA activates plasminogen directly (19).

A hypothetical mechanism of action explaining the apparent fibrin specificity of scu-PA in contrast to urokinase has been proposed (19) on the basis of the following observations:

1. In purified systems scu-PA activates plasminogen directly with a high affinity (low K_M), which compensates for the low turnover number (20). This high affinity is not mediated via the lysine-binding sites of plasminogen (63).
2. scu-PA does not significantly activate plasminogen in plasma in the absence of fibrin (63,64). Apparently a component in plasma competes with plasminogen for binding of scu-PA (19).
3. Following preincubation of scu-PA in plasma for up to 48 hr (18,64), efficient fibrinolysis without fibrinogenolysis is still observed following addition of a fibrin clot. Preliminary data suggest that the presence of fibrin reversed the inhibition execute by plasma, although direct binding of scu-PA to fibrin could not be demonstrated.

These findings suggest that the fibrin specificity of the activation of plasminogen by scu-PA is due to neutralization by fibrin of a component in plasma that competes with plasminogen for binding of scu-PA. The detailed molecular interactions that regulate the fibrin-specificity of scu-PA are not dependent on the amino-terminal and kringle-containing portions of the protein (62). The exact structure(s) responsible for its unique action, however, remain to be more precisely defined.

Inhibitors of Fibrinolysis

Two types of inhibitors have been recognized: those that inhibit plasmin (antiplasmins) and those that inhibit the activation of plasminogen (antiactivators). Human plasma exerts a very important inhibitory action on plasmin (65). For a long time it was accepted that there were essentially two functionally important plasmin inhibitors in plasma: an immediately reacting one and a slow-reacting one, identical with α_2-macroglobulin and α_1-antitrypsin, respectively (66). Later, however, a new plasmin inhibitor occurring in human plasma was described (67–70); this is now called α_2-antiplasmin. More recently, several inhibitors of t-PA and urokinase have been identified in plasma. A fast-acting inhibitor of t-PA and urokinase is relatively well characterized (46,48–50).

α_2-Antiplasmin

Physicochemical Properties. α_2-Antiplasmin is a glycoprotein composed of 452 amino acids containing four potential asparagine-based glycosylation sites (71). α_2-Antiplasmin is a member of the serine protease inhibitor family, which includes α_1-antitrypsin, angiotensinogen, antithrombin III, ovalbumin, α_1-antichymotrypsin, barley protein Z, mouse contrapsin, and C_1-esterase inhibitor.

The concentration of the inhibitor in normal plasma is about 7 mg/100 ml (about 1 μM) (68,72). α_2-Antiplasmin can be accurately determined in plasma, either with biological assays based on the very fast inhibition of plasmin and measurement of residual plasmin with natural or chromogenic substrates (73), or with immunological assays using specific antisera.

Already in the early purification procedure it was observed that the inhibitor in normal plasma was heterogeneous, consisting of functionally active and inactive material. Complete activation of the plasminogen present in normal plasma converted only about 0.7 of the antigen material into a complex with plasmin, while 0.3 of the inhibitor-related antigen appeared to be functionally inactive. Later work has shown that human plasma contains a form of the inhibitor that binds to plasminogen and one that does not bind (about 0.4 of the total), but still remains an active plasmin inhibitor (74). Both forms are immunochemically indistinguishable.

Mechanism of the Reaction with Plasmin. The inhibition of plasmin by α_2-antiplasmin occurs in two successive reactions (75,76): a very fast, reversible, second-order reaction followed by a slower, irreversible, first-order reaction. The second-order rate constant was found to be greater than 10^7 M^{-1}s^{-1} (76), which is among the fastest protein-protein reactions so far described. The first step of the reaction is clearly dependent on the presence of one or more free lysine binding sites and an active site in the plasmin molecule (75–77).

With the elucidation of the primary structure of α_2-antiplasmin (71), the structure of its reactive center has now been established to consist of Arg 364-Met 365, corresponding to the reactive site Met 358-Ser 359 in α_1-antitrypsin.

The Fast-Acting Inhibitor of t-PA and Urokinase

Recently, a specific rapid-reacting inhibitor of t-PA with M_r 40,000 to 50,000 has been identified in normal human plasma at low concentration or at a higher concentration in some pathological plasma samples. Chmielewska et al. (49) reported a content of t-PA inhibitor in plasma samples from healthy individuals of 0.6 $\pm$ 0.5 U/ml (1 unit determined as the amount that neutralizes 1 unit—5 ng, or about 0.06 pmol—of t-PA in 10 min). Elevated levels were found in a group of patients with suspected disturbance of the hemostatic system (3.8 ± 2.7 U/ml). Verheijen et al. (78) reported a fast-acting inhibitory capacity for t-PA of about 0.5 U/ml (0.1 pmol/ml). Juhan-Vague et al. (50) found less than 1 IU inhibitor in plasma in healthy individuals (1 IU determined as the amount that neutralizes 1 IU (10 ng) of t-PA in 5 min). Several laboratories have obtained evidence for the existence of a rapidly acting inhibitor of t-PA at higher levels in pathological plasma samples (49,50,79). In addition, inhibitors of t-PA have been identified in endothelial cell culture fluids (46), human platelets (80), and human placenta (81). In all cases, the inhibitor level was well below the plasma concentration of t-PA that has been achieved during pharmacological coronary thrombolysis (82). Thus, the inhibitor is an unlikely explanation for resistance to thrombolysis with t-PA, and at present, although the existence of a specific rapid inhibitor of t-PA in plasma has been clearly established, its exact pathophysiological role remains to be determined.

II. MECHANISM OF FIBRIN-SPECIFIC THROMBOLYSIS

Plasmin, the proteolytic enzyme of the fibrinolytic system, is a serine protease with a relatively low substrate specificity. In purified systems it will degrade fibrinogen as well as fibrin. When plasmin circulates freely in the blood, it will degrade a number of plasma proteins, including fibrinogen and the blood coagulation factors V and VIII.

Plasma does, however, contain a fast-acting plasmin inhibitor, α_2-antiplasmin, which reacts extremely rapidly with plasmin (76). Thus, small amounts of plasmin formed in the blood will be inhibited with a $t_{1/2}$ of 0.1 s. The rapidity of this reaction is dependent, however, on the availability of structures in the plasmin molecule called lysine-binding sites and on the availability of a free active site in the enzyme. Removal or saturation of the lysine-binding sites in plasmin will reduce the reaction rate with α_2-antiplasmin by a factor of 50, whereas low M_r substrates will compete with α_2-antiplasmin for the enzyme. Plasmin generated on the fibrin surface has both its lysine-binding sites and active site occupied and is therefore only slowly inactivated by α_2-antiplasmin. Plasmin generated in the circulating blood will rapidly be neutralized by α_2-antiplasmin. Excess circulating free plasmin activity will induce a systemic fibrinolytic state, characterized by degradation of fibrinogen and the blood coagulation factors V and VIII. Clot-specific thrombolysis will, in view of the interactions outlined above, require plasminogen activation at or in the vicinity of the fibrin clot.

One approach to obtaining specific thrombolysis is the use of thrombolytic agents that are stimulated by the presence of fibrin. Indeed, streptokinase and urokinase, which have no specific affinity for fibrin, activate circulating and fibrin-bound plasminogen relatively indiscriminately. Plasmin formed in the circulation is immediately neutralized by α_2-antiplasmin, and once the inhibitor is exhausted, several plasma proteins are degraded by plasmin (fibrinogen, factor V, factor VIII, etc.), thereby causing hemostatic breakdown.

The two physiological plasminogen activators t-PA and scu-PA exert a high degree of clot specificity in a plasma environment. This fibrin selectivity is regulated, however, by different molecular interactions.

Thrombolysis with t-PA

t-PA is relatively but not totally inactive in the absence of fibrin, and fibrin strikingly enhances the activation rate of plasminogen by t-PA (11). This is explained by an increased affinity of fibrin-bound t-PA for plasminogen and not by alteration of the catalytic efficiency of the enzyme. The kinetic data of Hoylaerts et al. (11) support a mechanism in which t-PA and plasminogen adsorb to a fibrin clot in a sequential and ordered way, yielding a cyclic ternary complex. Fibrin essentially increases the local plasminogen concentration by creating an additional interaction between t-PA and its substrate. The high affinity of t-PA for plasminogen in the presence of fibrin thus allows preferential activation on the fibrin clot.

The clot specificity of the activation of plasminogen by t-PA in vivo, however, is relative and not absolute. Thus, at the high infusion rates currently used to obtain rapid coronary artery reperfusion in patients with acute myocardial infarction (40 to 90 mg over 1 hr), the plasma level of t-PA is raised to approximately 1000 times the physiological concentration. Under these conditions, systemic activation of the fibrinolytic system occurs to a variable degree in vivo (82). In addition, in vitro activation following blood sampling occurs in the test tube if no specific precautions are taken (83).

Thrombolysis with scu-PA

The following hypothetical mechanism for the clot-specificity of scu-PA is compatible with our present findings (19,20). scu-PA has a much higher affinity for plasminogen ($K_M = 0.3$ μM) than does urokinase ($K_M = 25$ μM), but a lower catalytic rate constant ($k_{cat} = 0.02$ s^{-1} as compared to 1.0 s^{-1}). However, scu-PA does not activate plasminogen in plasma in the absence of a fibrin clot, due to the presence of a competitive inhibitor (20). Nevertheless, in a plasma milieu, specific clot lysis is obtained in the absence of systemic activation of the fibrinolytic system.

Preliminary data suggest that fibrin neutralizes the competitive inhibition, but this does not seem to occur via specific binding of scu-PA to fibrin. In contrast to t-PA, endogenous scu-PA (incorporated in a fibrin clot) does not have a higher thrombolytic activity in a clot lysis system than exogenous scu-PA.

Initial experience in patients with acute myocardial infarction (84,85) also has revealed that the fibrin specificity of thrombolysis with scu-PA is only relative. Thus, with infusion rates of 40 to 70 mg scu-PA over 1 hr, plasma levels rise to up to 5 μg/ml and extensive systemic fibrinolytic activation occurs in about 25% of the patients.

Synergism Between the Thrombolytic Properties of scu-PA and t-PA

Absence of In Vitro Synergism

A potential synergistic effect of t-PA and scu-PA or urokinase on clot lysis was investigated in a whole human plasma system in vitro (86). Combinations of t-PA and scu-PA, t-PA and urokinase, and scu-PA and urokinase at thrombolytic doses of each showed no synergism for thrombolysis.

In Vivo Synergism in Animals

In vivo, however, in a jugular vein thrombosis model in the rabbit, significant synergism between t-PA and scu-PA and between t-PA and urokinase on thrombolysis was observed (87). Intravenous infusion over 4 hr of t-PA, scu-PA, or urokinase, in amounts up to 0.5, 1.0, or 2.0 mg per kg body weight, resulted in significant thrombolysis (30 to 60%). The simultaneous infusion of t-PA and scu-PA or of t-PA and urokinase, but not of scu-PA and urokinase, had a significantly higher thrombolytic effect than could be anticipated on the basis of the added effects of each agent alone.

In Vivo Synergism in Man

Preliminary results in patients with acute myocardial infarction (88) suggest that t-PA and scu-PA, and t-PA and urokinase, may act synergistically in man as well. Intravenous infusion of 10 mg t-PA and 3 mg scu-PA over 60 min in three patients with acute myocardial infarction resulted in coronary reperfusion after 40 $\pm$ 14 min. Infusion of 10 mg t-PA and 300,000 IU urokinase in four patients produced coronary reperfusion in three of these patients in 46, 50, and 53 min, respectively. These doses are far lower than the currently used infusion rates of scu-PA or t-PA alone (40 to 80 mg over 1 hr). The combined infusions were not associated with systemic fibrinogen degradation. Trials with larger numbers of patients will be required to confirm these observations.

This demonstration of in vivo synergism contrasts with the lack of synergism in the in vitro clot lysis systems. Obviously, additional factors found only in vivo are involved. This is supported by the observation that the dose-response of in vivo thrombolysis with scu-PA is linear, whereas a clear threshold phenomenon of clot lysis in a plasma environment is observed in vitro. The confirmation of synergy between specific thrombolytic agents may permit a significant reduction of total administered doses, possibly with reduction or elimination of the systemic activation of the fibrinolytic system and concomitant fibrinogen breakdown.

III. CONCLUSIONS

Despite very significant progress in the understanding of the biochemistry and biological properties of thrombolytic agents over the last decade, thrombolytic therapy is not yet ingrained in current medical practice. Obvious reasons are the risk and unpredictability of bleeding and the uncertainty of the risk: benefit ratio with the currently available thrombolytic agents streptokinase and urokinase. New thrombolytic agents with better fibrin selectivity and, hopefully, better benefit:risk ratios are currently under clinical investigation. The first clinical trials with t-PA indicate that more effective thrombolysis can be obtained at a dose that induces less extensive systemic fibrinogenolysis than can be obtained with streptokinase. Further developments in this field may be expected.

REFERENCES

1. Sottrup-Jensen L, Petersen TE, Magnusson S: In *Atlas of Protein Sequence and Structure*, vol. 5, suppl. 3, Dayhoff MO, Ed., National Biochemical Research Foundation, Washington, D.C., 1978, p. 91.
2. Rabiner SF, Goldfine JD, Hart A, Summaria L, Robbins KC: Radioimmunoassay of human plasminogen and plasmin. J Lab Clin Med 74:265–274, 1969.
3. Friberger P, Knos M: Plasminogen determination in human plasma. In *Chromogenic Peptide Substrates*, Scully MF, Kakkar VV, Eds., Churchill Livingstone, Edinburgh, Scotland, 1979, pp. 128–140.
4. Deutsch DG, Mertz ET: Plasminogen: purification from human plasma by affinity chromatography. Science 170:1095–1096, 1970.

5. Robbins KC, Summaria L, Hsieh B, Shah RJ: The peptide chains of human plasmin. Mechanism of activation of human plasminogen to plasmin. J Biol Chem 242:2333–2342, 1967.

6. Groskopf WR, Summaria L, Robbins KC: Studies on the active center of human plasmin. Partial amino acid sequence of a peptide containing the active center serine residue. J Biol Chem 244:3590–3597, 1969.

7. Wiman B, Wallen P: Activation of human plasminogen by an insoluble derivative of urokinase. Structural changes of plasminogen in the course of activation to plasmin and demonstration of a possible intermediate compound. Eur J Biochem 36:25–31, 1973.

8. Holvoet P, Lijnen HR, Collen D: A monoclonal antibody specific for Lys-plasminogen. Application to the study of the activation pathways of plasminogen in vivo. J Biol Chem 260:12106–12111, 1985.

9. Wohl RC, Sinio L, Summaria L, Robbins KC: Comparative activation kinetics of mammalian plasminogen. Biochim Biophys Acta 745:20–31, 1983.

10. Christensen U, Müllertz S: Kinetic studies on the urokinase catalyzed conversion of NH_2-terminal lysine plasminogen to plasmin. Biochim Biophys Acta 480: 275–281, 1977.

11. Hoylaerts M, Rijken DC, Lijnen HR, Collen D: Kinetics of the activation of plasminogen by human tissue plasminogen activator. Role of fibrin. J Biol Chem 257:2912–2919, 1982.

12. Ranby M: Studies on the kinetics of plasminogen activation by tissue plasminogen activator. Biochim Biophys Acta 704:461–469, 1982.

13. Zamarron C, Lijnen HR, Collen D: Kinetics of the activation of plasminogen by natural and recombinant tissue-type plasminogen activator. J Biol Chem 259: 2080–2083, 1984.

14. Nieuwenhuizen W, Voskuilen M, Vermond A, Hoegee B, Traas DW, Verheijen JH: Kinetics of plasminogen activation by t-PA: the role of fibrinogen fragments. Haemostasis 14(abstr):71, 1984.

15. Suenson E, Lützen O, Thorsen S: Initial plasmin-degradation of fibrin as the basis of a positive feedback mechanism in fibrinolysis. Eur J Biochem 140:513–522, 1984.

16. Ranby M, Bergsdorf N, Norrman B, Suenson E, Wallen P: Tissue plasminogen activator kinetics. In *Progress in Fibrinolysis,* vol. 6, Davidson JF, Bachmann F, Bouvier CA, Kruithof EKO, Eds., Churchill Livingstone, Edinburgh, Scotland, 1983, pp. 182–184.

17. Rijken DC, Hoylaerts M, Collen D: Fibrinolytic properties of one-chain and two-chain human extrinsic (tissue-type) plasminogen activator. J Biol Chem 257:2920–2925, 1982.

18. Gurewich V, Pannell R, Louie S, Kelley P, Suddith RL, Greenlee R: Effective and fibrin-specific clot lysis by a zymogen precursor form of urokinase (pro-UK). A study in vitro and in two animal species. J Clin Invest 73:1731–1739, 1984.

19. Lijnen HR, Zamarron C, Blaber M, Winkler ME, Collen D: Activation of plasminogen by pro-urokinase. I. Mechanism. J Biol Chem 261:1253–1258, 1986.

20. Collen D, Zamarron C, Lijnen HR, Hoylaerts M: Activation of plasminogen by pro-urokinase. II. Kinetics. J Biol Chem 261:1259–1266, 1986.

21. Alkjaersig N: The purification and properties of human plasminogen. Biochem J 93:171–182, 1964.

22. Hoylaerts M, Lijnen HR, Collen D: Studies on the mechanism of the anti-fibrinolytic action of tranexamic acid. Biochim Biophys Acta 673:75–85, 1981.

23. Rickli EE, Otavsky WI: A new method of isolation and some properties of heavy chain of human plasmin. Eur J Biochem 9:441–447, 1975.

24. Wiman B, Lijnen HR, Collen D: On the specific interaction between the lysine-binding sites in plasmin and complementary sites in α_2-antiplasmin and in fibrinogen. Biochim Biophys Acta 579:142–159, 1979.

25. Thorsen S: Differences in the binding to fibrin of native plasminogen and plasminogen modified by proteolytic degradation. Influence of omega-amino-carboxylic acids. Biochim Biophys Acta 393:55–65, 1975.

26. Rakoczi I, Wiman B, Collen D: On the biological significance of the specific interaction between fibrin, plasminogen and antiplasmin. Biochim Biophys Acta 540:295–300, 1978.

27. Wiman B, Collen D: Molecular mechanism of physiological fibrinolysis. Nature (London) 272:549–550, 1978.

28. Ratnoff OD: The surface-mediated initiation of blood coagulation and related phenomena. In *Haemostasis: Biochemistry, Physiology, and Pathology,* Ogston D, Bennett B, Eds., John Wiley & Sons, London, 1977, pp. 25–55.

29. White WF, Barlow GH, Mozen MM: The isolation and characterization of plasminogen activators (urokinase) from human urine. Biochemistry 5:2160–2169, 1966.

30. Günzler WA, Steffens GJ, Otting F, Buse G, Flohe L: Structural relationship between human high and low molecular mass urokinase. Hoppe Seyler's Z Physiol Chem 363:133–141, 1982.

31. Günzler WA, Steffens GJ, Otting F, Kim SMA, Frankus E, Flohe L: The primary structure of high molecular mass urokinase from human urine. Hoppe-Seyler's Z Physiol Chem 363:1155–1165, 1982.

32. Heyneker HL, Holmes WE, Vehar GA: Preparation of functional human urokinase proteins, European Patent Application no. 83103629.8, publication no. 0092182A2, European Patent Office, Munich, Federal Republic of Germany, 1983.

33. Holmes WE, Pennica D, Blaber H, Rey MW, Günzler AW, Steffens GJ, Heyneker HL: Cloning and expression of the gene for pro-urokinase in *Escherichia coli.* Biotechnology 3:923–929, 1985.

34. Verstraete M: A far-reaching program: rapid, safe and predictable thrombolysis in man. In *Fibrinolysis,* Kline DL, Reddy NN, Eds., CRC Press, Boca Raton, Florida, 1980, pp. 129–149.

35. Müllertz S, Lassen M: An activator system in blood indispensable for the formation of plasmin by streptokinase. Proc Soc Exp Biol Med 82:264–268, 1953.

36. Kosow DP: Kinetic mechanism of the activation of human plasminogen by streptokinase. Biochemistry 14:4459–4465, 1975.

37. Gonzales-Gronow M, Siefring GE Jr, Castellino FJ: Mechanism of activation of human plasminogen by the activator complex, streptokinase-plasmin. J Biol Chem 253:1090–1094, 1978.

38. Pennica D, Holmes WE, Kohr WJ, Harkins RN, Vehar GA, Ward DA, Bennett WF, Yelverton E, Seeburg PH, Heyneker HL, Goeddel DV, Collen D: Cloning and expression of human tissue-type plasminogen activator cDNA in *E. coli.* Nature (London) 301:214–221, 1983.

39. Rijken DC, Collen D: Purification and characterization of the plasminogen activator secreted by human melanoma cells in culture. J Biol Chem 256:7035–7041, 1981.

40. Banyai L, Varadi A, Patthy L: Common evolutionary origin of the fibrin-binding structures of fibronectin and tissue-type plasminogen activator. FEBS Lett 163:37–41, 1983.

41. Ny T, Backman A, Elgh F, Enquist K, Fredrikson C, Jarvinen S: Isolation and characterization of the genomic region carrying the human tissue plasminogen activator gene. Haemostasis 14(abstr):56, 1984.

42. Ranby M, Bergsdorf N, Nilsson T: Enzymatic properties of one-chain and two-chain forms of tissue plasminogen activator. Thromb Res 27:175–183, 1982.

43. Loskutoff DJ, Edgington T: Synthesis of a fibrinolytic activator and inhibitor by endothelial cells. Proc Nat Acad Sci USA 74:3903–3907, 1977.

44. Levin EG, Loskutoff DJ: Cultured bovine endothelial cells produce both urokinase and tissue-type plasminogen activators. J Cell Biol 94:631–636, 1983.

45. Rijken DC, Wijngaards G, Welbergen J: Relationship between tissue plasminogen activator and the activators in blood and vascular wall. Thromb Res 18:815–830, 1980.

46. Loskutoff DJ, Van Mourik JA, Erickson LA, Lawrence D: Detection of an unusually stable fibrinolytic inhibitor produced by bovine endothelial cells. Proc Nat Acad Sci 80:2956–2960, 1984.

47. Christensen U, Holmberg L, Bladh B, Astedt B: Kinetics between urokinase and an inhibitor of fibrinolysis from placental tissue. Thromb Haemost 48:24–26, 1982.

48. Kruithof EK, Ransijn A, Bachmann F: Inhibition of tissue plasminogen activator by human plasma. In *Progress in Fibrinolysis,* vol. VI, Davidson JF, Bachmann F, Bouvier CA, Kruithof EKO, Eds., Churchill Livingstone, Edinburgh, Scotland, 1983, pp. 362–366.

49. Chmielewska J, Ranby M, Wiman B: Evidence for a rapid inhibitor to tissue plasminogen activator in plasma. Thromb Res 31:427–436, 1983.

50. Juhan-Vague I, Moerman B, De Cock F, Aillaud MF, Collen D: Plasma levels of a specific inhibitor of tissue-type plasminogen activator (and urokinase) in normal and pathological conditions. Thromb Res 33:523–530, 1984.

51. Korninger C, Stassen JM, Collen D: Turnover of human extrinsic (tissue-type) plasminogen activator in rabbits. Thromb Haemost 46:658–661, 1981.

52. Holvoet P, Lijnen HR, Collen D: Characterization of functional domains in human tissue-type plasminogen activator with the use of monoclonal antibodies. Eur J Biochem 158:173–177, 1986.

53. Bernik MB: Increased plasminogen activator (urokinase) in tissue culture after fibrin deposition. J Clin Invest 52:823–834, 1973.

54. Nolan C, Hall L, Barlow G, Tribby IIE: Plasminogen activator from human embryonic kidney cell cultures: Evidence for a proactivator. Biochim Biophys Acta 496:384–400, 1977.

55. Husain S, Gurewich V, Lipinski B: Purification and partial characterization of a single-chain high-molecular-weight form of urokinase from human urine. Arch Biochim Biophys 220:31–38, 1983.

56. Stump DC, Thienpont M, Collen D: Urokinase-related proteins in human urine. Isolation and characterization of single-chain urokinase (pro-urokinase) and uro-kinase-inhibitor complex. J Biol Chem 261:1267–1273, 1986.

57. Wun TC, Schleuning WD, Reich E: Isolation and characterization of urokinase from human plasma. J Biol Chem 257:3276–3283, 1982.

58. Sumi H, Maruyama M, Matsuo O, Mihara H, Toki N: Higher fibrin-binding and thrombolytic properties of single polypeptide chain-high molecular weight uro-kinase. Thromb Haemost 47:297, 1982.

59. Kohno T, Hopper P, Lillquist JS, Suddith RL, Greenlee R, Moir DT: Kidney plasminogen activator: a precursor form of human urokinase with high fibrin affinity. Biotechnology 2:628–635, 1984.

60. Kasai S, Arimura H, Nishida M, Suyama T: Proteolytic cleavage of single-chain pro-urokinase induces conformational change which follows activation of the zymogen and reduction of its high affinity for fibrin. J Biol Chem 260:12377–12381, 1985.

61. Stump DC, Lijnen HR, Collen D: Purification and characterization of single-chain urokinase-type plasminogen activator (scu-PA) from human cell cultures. J Biol Chem 261:1274–1278, 1986.

62. Stump DC, Lijnen HR, Collen D: Purification and characterization of a novel low molecular weight form of single chain urokinase-type plasminogen activator (submitted).

63. Lijnen HR, Zamarron C, Collen D: Characterization of the high-affinity interaction between human plasminogen and pro-urokinase. Eur J Biochem 150:141–144, 1985.

64. Zamarron C, Lijnen HR, Van Hoef B, Collen D: Biological and thrombolytic properties of proenzyme and active forms of urokinase. I. Fibrinolytic and fibrinogenolytic properties in human plasma in vitro of urokinases obtained from human urine or by recombinant DNA technology. Thromb Haemost 52:19–23, 1984.

65. Norman PS: Studies of the plasmin system. II. Inhibition of plasmin by serum or plasma. J Exp Med 108:53–68, 1958.

66. Schwick HG, Heimburger N, Haupt H: Antiproteasen des Humanserums. Z Inn Med 21:1–6, 1966.

67. Collen D: Identification and some properties of a new fast-reacting plasmin inhibitor in human plasma. Eur J Biochem 69:209–216, 1976.

68. Moroi M, Aoki N: Isolation and characterization of α_2-plasmin inhibitor from human plasma. A novel proteinase inhibitor which inhibits activator-induced clot lysis. J Biol Chem 251:5956–5965, 1976.

69. Müllertz S, Clemmensen I: The primary inhibitor of plasmin in human plasma. Biochem J 159:545–553, 1976.

70. Bagge L, Bjork I, Saldeen T, Wallin R: Purification and characterization of an inhibitor of plasminogen activation from posttraumatic patients. Forensic Sci 7:83–86, 1976.

71. Holmes WE, Nelles L, Lijnen HR, Collen D: Primary structure of human α_2-antiplasmin, a serine protease inhibitor (serpin). J Biol Chem (in press).

72. Wiman B, Collen D: Purification and characterization of human antiplasmin, the fast-acting plasmin inhibitor in plasma. Eur J Biochem 78:19–26, 1977.

73. Edy J, De Cock F, Collen D: Inhibition of plasmin by normal and antiplasmin-depleted human plasma. Thromb Res 8:513–518, 1976.

74. Christensen U, Clemmensen I: Purification and reaction mechanisms of the primary inhibitor of plasmin from human plasma. Biochem J 175:635–641, 1978.

75. Christensen U, Clemmensen I: Kinetic properties of the primary inhibitor of plasmin from human plasma. Biochem J 163:389–391, 1977.

76. Wiman B, Collen D: On the kinetics of the reaction between human antiplasmin and plasmin. Eur J Biochem 84:573–578, 1978.

77. Wiman B, Boman L, Collen D: On the kinetics of the reaction between human antiplasmin and a low-molecular weight form of plasmin. Eur J Biochem 87:143–146, 1978.

78. Verheijen JH, Chang GIC, Kluft C: Evidence for the occurrence of a fast-acting inhibitor for tissue-type plasminogen activator in human plasma. Thromb Haemost 51:392–395, 1984.

79. Wijngaards G, Groeneveld E: Temporarily increased inhibition by plasma of plasminogen activator activity in severely ill patients. Haemostasis 12(abstr 188):571, 1982.

80. Erickson LA, Ginsberg MH, Loskutoff DJ: Detection and partial characterization of an inhibitor of plasminogen activator in human platelets. J Clin Invest 74:1465–1472, 1984.

81. Astedt B, Lecander I, Broden T, Lundblad A, Löw K: Purification of a specific placental plasminogen activator inhibitor by monoclonal antibody and its complex formation with plasminogen activator. Thromb Haemost 53:122, 1985.

82. Collen D, Bounameaux H, De Cock F, Lijnen HR, Verstraete M: Analysis of coagulation and fibrinolysis during intravenous infusion of recombinant human tissue-type plasminogen activator (t-PA) in patients with acute myocardial infarction. Circulation 73:511–517, 1986.

83. Holvoet P, Lijnen HR, Collen D: A monoclonal antibody preventing binding of tissue-type plasminogen activator (t-PA) to fibrin, useful to monitor fibrinogen breakdown during t-PA infusion. Blood 67:1482–1487, 1986.
84. Van de Werf F, Nobuhara M, Collen D: Coronary thrombolysis with human single chain urokinase-type plasminogen activator (scu-PA) in patients with acute myocardial infarction. Ann Int Med 104:345–348, 1986.
85. Van de Werf F, Vanhaecke J, De Geest H, Verstraete M, Collen D: Coronary thrombolysis with recombinant single chain urokinase-type plasminogen activator (rscu-PA) in patients with acute myocardial infarction. Circulation 74:1066–1070, 1986.
86. Collen D, De Cock F, Demarsin E, Lijnen HR, Stump DC: Absence of synergism between tissue-type plasminogen activator (t-PA), single chain urokinase-type plasminogen activator (scu-PA), and urokinase on clot lysis in a plasma milieu in vitro. Thromb Haemost 56:35–39, 1986.
87. Collen D, Stassen JM, Stump DC, Verstraete M: In vivo synergism of thrombolytic agents. Circulation 74:838–842, 1986.
88. Collen D, Stump DC, Van de Werf F: Coronary thrombolysis in patients with acute myocardial infarction by intravenous infusion of synergic thrombolytic agents. Am Heart J 112:1083–1084, 1986.

2

Pharmacodynamics of Activation of Plasminogen with t-PA

Alan J. Tiefenbrunn and Burton E. Sobel
Washington University School of Medicine
St. Louis, Missouri

I. INTRODUCTION

A major pharmacological attribute of tissue-type plasminogen activator (t-PA) is its relatively high affinity for fibrin. This property facilitates its interaction with plasminogen bound to fibrin (1), as indicated by the kinetics of the reactions depicted in Table 1. The apparent Michaelis constant (K_M) for each of the reactions is indicated. The low K_M of 0.14 μM characterizing the activation of plasminogen bound to fibrin implies that this reaction will be kinetically favored over activation of free plasminogen whenever concentrations of t-PA are relatively low. The differing kinetic features of interaction of t-PA with fibrin-bound compared with free plasminogen give rise to localized formation of plasmin within and on nascent thrombi and dissolution of fibrin clots without substantial plasminemia and the associated degradation of circulating fibrinogen and other plasma proteins. Thus, "clot selectivity" of t-PA is a function of fundamental biochemical properties of components of the fibrinolytic system. Selectivity also reflects the intensity and duration of exposure of plasminogen to activator in the domain of fibrin compared with plasminogen in the systemic circulation.

The kinetics of reactions participating in fibrinolysis can be characterized quantitatively. We have developed a physiologically based mathematical model designed to characterize interactions among the integrated biochemical

Table 1   Reactions Involved in Activation of Plasminogen by t-PA in the Circulation and on Fibrin Clots

---

In plasma

$$\text{t-PA} + \text{plasminogen} \underset{k_{-1}}{\overset{k_1}{\rightleftharpoons}} [\text{t-PA} \cdot \text{plasminogen}] \overset{k_2}{\rightarrow} \text{t-PA} + \text{plasmin}$$

$$\frac{k_{-1}}{k_1} = K_M{}^a = 65 \ \mu M$$

In fibrin

$$\text{t-PA} + [\text{plasminogen} \cdot \text{fibrin}] \underset{k_{-3}}{\overset{k_3}{\rightleftharpoons}} [\text{t-PA} \cdot \text{plasminogen} \cdot \text{fibrin}] \overset{k_4}{\rightarrow} [\text{t-PA} \cdot \text{plasmin} \cdot \text{fibrin}]$$

$$\frac{k_{-3}}{k_3} = K_M = 0.14 \ \mu M$$

---

[a]Michaelis constant.
Brackets surrounding two or more constituents joined by a dot symbolize a complex.
k_x and k_{-x} refer to forward and reverse rate constants, respectively.

reactions known to be involved in fibrinolysis as a function of time, prevailing concentrations of t-PA, and concentrations of other constituents of the fibrinolytic system. The model has been used for computer-assisted simulation and prediction of pharmacodynamics of t-PA administered in conformity with a wide variety of dose regimens. It has been particularly useful for elucidating the safety and efficacy of t-PA in comparison with those of other activators and as a function of dose and duration of administration. It has been helpful also for delineating effects of dose regimens selected to conform to individual characteristics of patients and to specific therapeutic objectives.

Some examples reflecting the diversity of clinical considerations relevant to thrombolysis merit consideration. One is represented by a patient with acute myocardial infarction attributable to a thrombus occluding a coronary artery. The clot may be quite small. However, it must be lysed very rapidly because the extent of myocardial infarction increases with each minute of ischemia. In fact, hope of significant salvage of myocardium becomes vanishingly small after ischemia has persisted for only a few hours. For such a patient, the dose of activator must be high. However, only a short-term initial infusion of t-PA may be needed.

In contrast, a patient presenting with extensive deep vein thrombosis may have a volume of clot several orders of magnitude greater than that present with evolving myocardial infarction. Clot dissolution is needed to diminish the risk of pulmonary embolism and to improve the likelihood of long-term competence of venous valves. However, the rate of dissolution is not as critical as it is for patients with coronary thrombi. With deep venous thrombosis, prolonged infusions of t-PA or repeated infusions over several days may be required. Prospective characterization of expected effects and relative safety of thrombolytic agents applied in such diverse clinical applications is needed.

Computer simulation of consequences of reactions involved in fibrinolysis and their multiple biochemical constituents has provided insight regarding the relative importance of individual reactions, the forward and reverse rate constants of each, and the influence of changes in prevailing concentrations of the biochemical moieties involved.

II. ACTIVATION OF FIBRINOLYSIS

The hemostatic and fibrinolytic systems have been characterized extensively with respect to component proteins, their physiological concentrations in plasma, and the kinetics of participating biochemical reactions and their interactions. Although accurate assay of constituents is sometimes demanding, conventional assay procedures are sensitive and specific. Thus, predictions regarding pharmacodynamics of t-PA can be correlated with observed changes of concentrations of plasma proteins (2).

Clinically available activators of fibrinolysis act by directly or indirectly activating plasminogen. None has intrinsic fibrinolytic activity. Plasminogen is a circulating glycoprotein with a high affinity for fibrin (3). Activation to yield plasmin involves peptide bond cleavage. Plasmin is a serine protease capable of degrading fibrinogen and other coagulation factors as well as fibrin. Thus, elaboration of excess plasmin in the circulation can be detrimental. Prolonged impairment of hemostasis can result because of consumption of clotting factors and generation of high concentrations of fibrinogen degradation products that inhibit clot formation and platelet function. Physiologically, protection from excess plasmin in the circulation is conferred by its rapid inactivation by circulating α_2-antiplasmin. However, pharmacological doses of activators of fibrinolysis can deplete α_2-antiplasmin, which is consumed when it interacts with the massive amounts of plasmin that may be generated.

α_2-Antiplasmin is a rapidly acting inhibitor of plasmin. Its inhibition dominates under physiological conditions. α_2-Antiplasmin contributes to the rapid neutralization and perhaps clearance of circulating plasmin, thereby preventing nonspecific proteolysis. Other inhibitors of plasmin exist, including α_2-macroglobulin, a large circulating protein capable of trapping plasmin as well as other serine proteases and blocking their proteolytic activity. The reaction of α_2-macroglobulin with plasmin is relatively slow and may not be of great importance under physiological circumstances. However, under conditions of pharmacological activation of plasminogen and depletion of circulating α_2-antiplasmin, the reaction becomes very important.

In addition to the reactions shown in Table 1, several reactions influence effects of t-PA administered pharmacologically on generation of plasmin in the circulation. Some are shown in Table 2. The effects of plasmin acting on a fibrin surface are quantitatively small with respect to constituents in the circulating blood and do not affect overall hemostatic competence. Physiologically circulating inhibitors of t-PA such as the so-called fast inhibitor can be disregarded when t-PA is used in pharmacological doses because their concentrations are negligible in comparison with those of the administered t-PA. Induction of high levels of inhibitors is a theoretical possibility, however, and could lead to rebound impairment of fibrinolysis. Inactivation or breakdown of t-PA in plasma or in the liver can be compensated for by continuous intravenous infusion that will maintain virtually constant plasma t-PA levels. Plasma levels of t-PA are proportional to infusion rate (4). For purposes of comparison, approximate plasma t-PA levels that can be anticipated with some selected treatment regimens are shown in Table 3.

Table 2   Reactions Involving Plasmin in the Circulation

$$\text{Plasmin} + \alpha_2\text{-antiplasmin} \underset{k_{-5}}{\overset{k_5}{\rightleftharpoons}} [\text{Plasmin} \cdot \alpha_2\text{-antiplasmin}]$$

$$[\text{Plasmin} \cdot \alpha_2\text{-antiplasmin}] \overset{k_6}{\longrightarrow} \text{Inactive fragments}$$

$$\text{Plasmin} + \text{fibrinogen} \underset{k_{-7}}{\overset{k_7}{\rightleftharpoons}} [\text{Plasmin} \cdot \text{fibrinogen}]$$

$$[\text{Plasmin} \cdot \text{fibrinogen}] \overset{k_8}{\longrightarrow} \text{Plasmin} + \text{FDPs}^a$$

$$\text{Plasmin} + \alpha_2\text{-macroglobulin} \overset{k_9}{\longrightarrow} [\text{Plasmin} \cdot \alpha_2\text{-macroglobulin}]$$

---

[a]Fibrinogen degradation products.
Brackets surrounding two constituents joined by a dot symbolize a complex.
k_x and k_{-x} refer to forward and reverse rate constants, respectively.

Table 3   Approximate Steady-State Plasma t-PA Levels Associated with Selected Intravenous Infusion Regimens

Condition	Dose of t-PA (normalized for 80-kg patient)			Concentration of t-PA		
	mg/hr	mg/kg/hr	μg/kg/min	ng/ml	nM	μM
Physiological	—	—	—	6	0.1	0.0001
Treatment of MI (1986)[a]	80	1	16.7	6000	100	0.10
Treatment of MI (1984)[b]	40	0.5	8.3	3000	50	0.05
"Maintenance" after clot lysis (1986)[a]	10	0.125	2.1	750	12.5	0.0125
Treatment of PVD[c]	5	0.062	1.0	375	6.2	0.0062

[a]Dose for the Thrombolysis in Myocardial Infarction II (TIMI-II) trial was 90 mg over 1 hr followed by 10 mg/hr for 6 hr. MI = Myocardial infarction.
[b]Ref. 7.
[c]Ref. 6. PVD = Peripheral vascular disease (arterial occlusion).

III. COMPUTER SIMULATION

A Computer-Assisted Model

We have performed automated simulations of pharmacodynamic effects of infusion of t-PA with the use of a VAX 11/780 computer with software (KINSIM) kindly provided by Dr. Carl Frieden (5). KINSIM permits compilation of a series of as many as 40 chemical reactions, each of which can be represented by a chemical equation in standard format with defined forward and reverse rate constants or rapid equilibrium conditions. Parameters that can be specified by the operator include initial (or constant) concentrations of chemical constituents, values for each of the rate constants, intervals over which the reactions proceed, and scale factors for selected output. The program provides continuous solutions for the interactive differential chemical equations involved by numerical integration and calculation of derivatives at each selected time point to estimate concentrations of each component. Display options include lists of output values, CRT displays, and hard-copy plots.

Assumptions

Quantitative modeling of the biochemical reactions that accompany administration of t-PA requires several simplifications and assumptions (1,2):

1. The concentration of t-PA in the circulation can be measured accurately or estimated correctly from a standard dose response curve. In its simplest form, the model we have developed assumes a steady-state concentration of t-PA maintained by continuous intravenous infusion. The model can be applied as well to changing blood levels of t-PA such as those seen with intermittent dosing.
2. The rate constants for the reactions involved in vivo are similar to those determined with purified proteins in vitro.
3. The starting concentrations of components of the hemostatic and fibrinolytic systems at the onset of administration of t-PA are known. This assumption is difficult to fulfill. The relative and absolute concentrations of components are species-specific and vary with physiological stress such as bleeding or other trauma.
4. The systemic consequences of binding of t-PA to fibrin, activation of fibrin-bound plasminogen, and dissolution of fibrin within the clot are quantitatively negligible.
5. The effects of physiological circulating inhibitors of t-PA can be disregarded because inhibitors are overwhelmed by the high concentrations of t-PA associated with pharmacological doses.
6. Synthesis and release into the circulation of constituent plasma proteins require consideration only for relatively prolonged infusions of t-PA.
7. Values obtained in vitro in samples acquired from patients given activators of fibrinolysis accurately reflect events in vivo. This assumption and its limitations are considered below.

Reactions Included in the Model Developed

In addition to the activation of plasminogen by t-PA designated in Table 1, several reactions involving subsequent interactions of plasmin are summarized in Table 2. For short-term, high-dose infusions of t-PA, such as those used for treatment of patients with evolving myocardial infarction, synthesis and release into the circulation of plasma proteins, including plasminogen or fibrinogen, are too slow to be quantitatively important for predicting pharmacodynamic effects. However, for longer infusions lasting several hours such as those used in the treatment of peripheral arterial thrombosis (6), repletion of plasminogen must be considered and is included in our simulations. For very prolonged infusions (lasting more than approximately 12 hr) such as those required for treatment of deep venous thrombosis, repletion of fibrinogen, α_2-antiplasmin, and α_2-macroglobulin must be incorporated into simulations as well. Hepatic clearance of fibrinogen degradation products,

Table 4   Concentrations in Plasma of
Proteins Before Administration of t-PA

Constituent	Concentration (μM)
Fibrinogen	10
Plasminogen	2
α_2-Antiplasmin	1
α_2-Macroglobulin	3

Source: Ref. 2.

although relatively slow, may require simulation for evaluation of very prolonged infusions.

We assume that the concentrations in plasma of plasmin and fibrinogen degradation products are negligible at the time of onset of infusion of t-PA. Initial concentrations of plasma proteins as indicated in Table 4. The rate constants for the reactions involved are shown in Table 5 with subscripts corresponding to the reactions as numbered in Tables 1 and 2.

Table 5   Rate Constants of Reactions
Included in Simulations of Effects of Infusion
of t-PA

Constant	Value (per s)
k_1	10 μM^{-1}
k_{-1}	280
k_2	0.3
k_5	30 μM^{-1}
k_{-5}	0.0063
k_6	0.004
k_7	10 μM^{-1}
k_{-7}	300
k_8	25
k_9	0.35 μM^{-1}

Source: Ref. 2.

IV. VALIDATION OF THE RESULTS OF COMPUTER SIMULATIONS

Importance of α_2-Macroglobulin

One of the first phenomena to become evident during our initial simulations of pharmacodynamic effects of administration of t-PA was the importance of interaction of plasmin with an inhibitor other than α_2-antiplasmin, hypothetically α_2-macroglobulin. Measured plasma concentrations of α_2-antiplasmin rapidly approach zero with even moderate doses of t-PA given over 1 to 2 hr, as correctly predicted by the model. However, measured concentrations of circulating fibrinogen do not decline abruptly or markedly (7), even though our initial simulation implied that they would (Figure 1A). Thus, the model was modified to include an additional interaction that apparently becomes strikingly important when α_2-antiplasmin has been consumed. When an interaction between plasmin and α_2-macroglobulin and an association constant consistent with the known properties of α_2-macroglobulin were included in simulations, marked fibrinogenolysis was not predicted despite consumption of α_2-antiplasmin. The "protection" provided by circulating α_2-macroglobulin appears to account for the improved concordance between observed and simulated changes (Figure 1B).

Contributions of Protein Synthesis

Our early simulations overestimated the depletion of plasminogen in response to t-PA administered over several hours. This disparity was obviated by introducing a reaction that accounted for synthesis and release into the circulation of plasminogen, known to be relatively rapid judging from observations of changes in vivo. Thus, the half-time of recovery of plasma plasminogen after its nadir is approximately 12 hr (2).

Clinical Observations

Correlation of simulated changes of concentrations of plasma proteins with those measured in response to administration of thrombolytic agents requires that values determined in vitro be valid reflections of prevailing concentrations in vivo at the time of acquisition of blood samples. Unfortunately, however, activation of plasminogen may occur in vitro in samples containing pharmacological concentrations of t-PA or other activators. Such activation leads to degradation of fibrinogen and other proteins in the sample by plasmin generated in vitro. Artifact of this type is particularly likely in samples obtained early after bolus injections of activator or when high plasma levels of

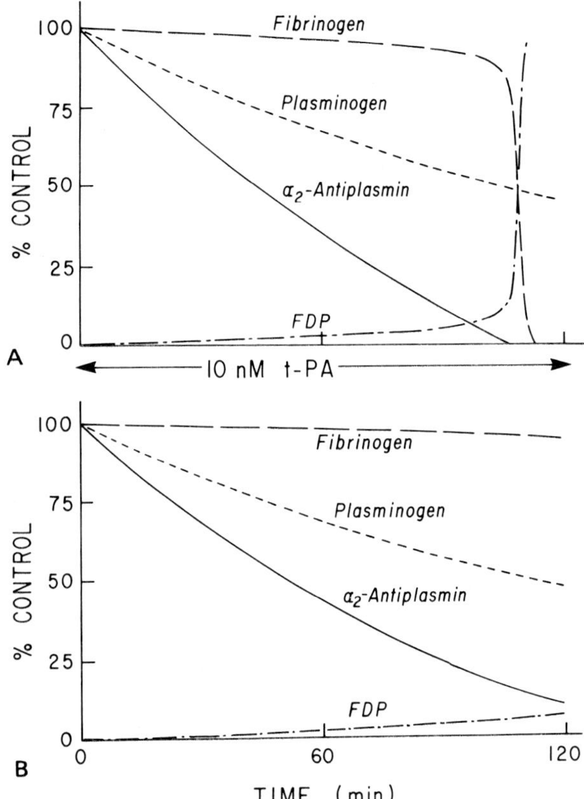

Figure 1 Simulations of serial changes in plasma constituents designated during infusion of t-PA sufficient to maintain the concentration of plasma t-PA at 10 nM for 2 hr. (A) Results under conditions in which reactions of plasmin with α_2-macroglobulin are neglected. Once α_2-antiplasmin has been consumed, profound fibrinogenolysis ensues. FDPs are expressed as percentages of baseline fibrinogen. (B) Results under conditions in which the interactions between plasmin and α_2-macroglobulin are considered. A modest reduction in the rate of consumption of α_2-antiplasmin occurs compared with that in panel A because of the interaction of plasmin with α_2-macroglobulin. However, even when consumption of α_2-antiplasmin is almost complete, marked fibrinogenolysis does not occur because of the interaction of plasmin being formed with α_2-macroglobulin. (From Ref. 2.)

activator have been reached in vivo during the course of infusions. Conventional approaches designed to preclude activation of plasmin in vitro entail prompt freezing and supplementation of samples of aprotinin, a serine protease inhibitor. However, they are of only limited value. Accordingly, we have employed another inhibitor of serine proteases, D-phenylalanyl-L-prolyl-L-arginine chloromethyl ketone · 2HCl (PPACK) and found it to effectively inhibit proteolysis and activation of plasminogen in vitro without distorting results of assay of plasminogen, α_2-antiplasmin, fibrinogen, or fibrinogen degradation products under specifically defined conditions (2). Supplementation of samples with this agent yielded close correlations between simulated values and observed results in patients. Figure 2 compares observed changes in plasma concentrations of fibrinogen and plasminogen in samples from one patient given 25 mg of t-PA over a 7-hr interval for treatment of peripheral arterial thrombosis. Activation of plasminogen in vivo was re-

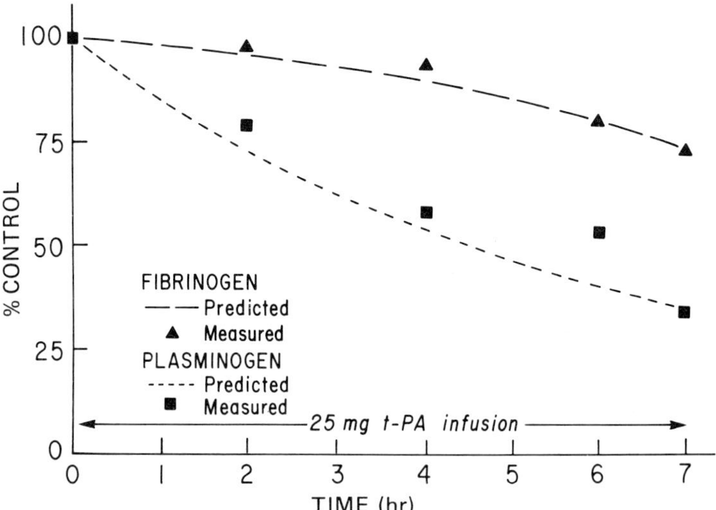

Figure 2   Comparisons of observed values for fibrinogen and plasminogen with those simulated for a patient given 25 mg of t-PA by continuous infusion for 7 hr. Values are percentages of concentrations present immediately before the onset of the infusion. Although samples were not protected with PPACK in this example, the prevailing concentrations of t-PA were low. Thus, marked fibrinogenolysis in vitro would be less likely to occur than it would in samples from patients given high doses of t-PA, such as those used for treatment of coronary thrombosis. (From Ref. 2.)

flected by the decrease in measured levels of plasminogen over the course of the infusion. A more modest decrease in the level of circulating fibrinogen was observed. Predicted and observed values for each of the two moieties correlated closely.

Similar concordance between predicted and observed values for the concentrations of fibrinogen and plasminogen was seen when results were analyzed from 101 patients in the European cooperative trial of t-PA for treatment of acute myocardial infarction (8). Patients in this study had been given 60 mg of t-PA over 90 min. Predicted concentrations of fibrinogen after 90 min of infusion were 73% of baseline. Observed values averaged 69 ± 3% (SE) of baseline. Predicted values for plasminogen at corresponding intervals were 33%. Observed values averaged 39 ± 4%, again quite concordant with estimates from the simulations.

Similar concordance was observed also between predictions from simulations and results from Phase I of the Thrombolysis in Myocardial Infarction (TIMI) trial of t-PA (9). Patients in the TIMI trial had been given 40 mg of t-PA intravenously over 1 hr followed by 20 mg/hr for 2 hr. Measured concentrations of fibrinogen at the end of the 3-hr infusions averaged 70 ± 16% (SD) of baseline (n = 32). Values agreed within 2% with estimates predicted from simulations of pharmacodynamics, assuming corresponding blood levels of t-PA maintained for the same interval.

V. IMPLICATIONS OF THE MODEL

As noted previously, the contributions of α_2-macroglobulin to pharmacodynamics is substantial, as are effects of synthesis and release into the circulation of plasminogen. When these effects were incorporated in simulations, prediction of effects of selected disparate regimens of infusion of t-PA could be made with reasonable confidence. Figure 3A illustrates the magnitude of depletion of plasminogen anticipated with selected blood levels of t-PA maintained for 1 hr compared with effects of the same concentrations maintained for 4 hr. Maintenance of a modest, pharmacological plasma concentration of t-PA (less than 10 nM) is anticipated to elicit only moderate depletion of plasminogen to approximately 70% of baseline. However, maintenance of a plasma concentration of t-PA of 10 nM for 4 hr is anticipated to elicit substantial depletion of plasminogen because of activation to plasmin with a consequent value of only 20% of baseline at the end of the hypothetical infusion. With higher blood levels of t-PA, approaching 100 nM, even a 1-hr infusion is anticipated to elicit profound depletion of plasminogen.

Figure 3B illustrates changes in concentrations of fibrinogen in plasma

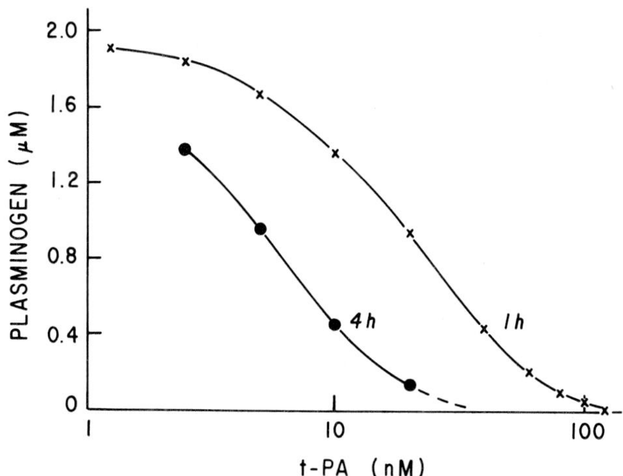

Figure 3A   Simulated concentrations of plasminogen in plasma (plotted on the ordinate) as a function of prevailing concentrations of t-PA throughout infusions for 1 or 4 hr. t-PA values on the abscissa are plotted on a logarithmic scale. The simulation indicates marked diminution of plasma plasminogen at the end of a 4-hr infusion even when plasma concentrations of t-PA do not exceed 10 nM. On the other hand, anticipated diminution of plasminogen is only modest at the end of a 1-hr infusion with a plasma concentration of this magnitude. Conversely, even a brief infusion of 1 hr is anticipated to lead to marked depletion of plasma plasminogen when the prevailing concentration of t-PA approaches 100 nM. (From Ref. 2.)

anticipated with selected blood levels of t-PA maintained for 1 hr. In spite of considerable activation of plasminogen with a concentration of t-PA of approximately 10 nM, depletion of fibrinogen is anticipated to be only minimal. The apparent protection of homeostasis is afforded by circulating α_2-antiplasmin and α_2-macroglobulin. However, with higher blood levels of t-PA, approaching 100 nM, depletion of fibrinogen is anticipated to be considerable. Thus, clot selectivity of t-PA is clearly relative rather than absolute.

It is apparent from the simulations that depletion of plasminogen results in a paradoxical and decreasing rate of depletion of fibrinogen. As can be seen from the curves in Figure 3, depletion of fibrinogen approaches an asymptote when depletion of plasminogen is profound because additional generation of plasmin is precluded. Under such conditions, administration of t-PA would not elicit formation of additional plasmin. Thus, acceleration of fibrinogen-

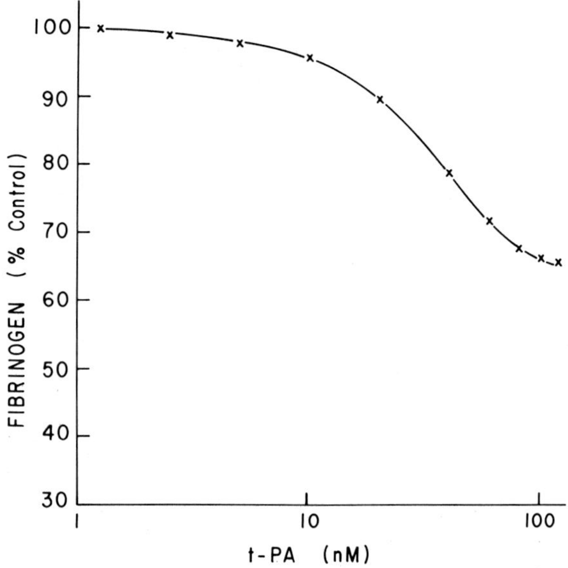

Figure 3B   Plasma fibrinogen (percentage of control) simulated as a function of the prevailing concentration of t-PA throughout a 1-hr infusion. Plasma t-PA concentrations on the abscissa are plotted on a logarithmic scale. Simulated depletion of fibrinogen reaches a limiting value despite hypothetically increasing concentrations of plasma t-PA throughout the 1-hr infusions. This phenomenon reflects the consumption of plasminogen and hence the paradoxical lack of generation of plasmin in the circulation when maintained concentrations of t-PA in plasma approach 100 nM. (From Ref. 2.)

olysis would not be anticipated. Knowledge of this paradox is important with respect to pharmacodynamic effects of prolonged infusions of t-PA. With such infusions, continued generation of plasmin ultimately becomes dependent on synthesis and release into the circulation of plasminogen from the liver. Because therapeutic effects of all available activators of the fibrinolytic system reflect activation of plasminogen, they become blunted when concentrations of plasminogen decline to values near zero. However, at the surface and in the interstices of a clot, plasminogen bound to fibrin may persist even when circulating plasminogen is markedly depleted because of the high affinity of plasminogen for fibrin. Furthermore, fibrin-bound, locally generated plasmin may persist on and within a clot because of its relative inaccessability to α_2-antiplasmin. Lysine binding sites of plasmin are involved in both interactions (with fibrin and α_2-antiplasmin). When occupied because of binding of plasminogen to fibrin, they are not available for interaction with α_2-antiplasmin (3). In view of these considerations, prolonged treatment with t-PA may be achieved best with intermittent dosing rather than continuous infusions of modest amounts of the agent that lead to consequent depletion of circulating plasminogen.

VI. SUMMARY

Simulations of the biochemical reactions involved in fibrinogenolysis and fibrinolysis and their interactions have been employed to characterize anticipated pharmacodynamic effects of administration of t-PA in disparate, selected dose regimens. Sequential changes of concentrations of plasma components of the hemostatic and fibrinolytic systems anticipated from simulations conform closely to observed changes under diverse clinical conditions. The importance of α_2-macroglobulin as an inhibitor of plasmin when circulating α_2-antiplasmin has been consumed is underscored, as is the importance of synthesis and release into the circulation of plasminogen and other proteins during prolonged infusions of t-PA. The relative as opposed to absolute clot selectivity of t-PA is emphasized as well. When activation of plasminogen becomes profound as a result of prolonged administration or use of excessively high doses of t-PA, fibrinogenolysis as well as fibrinolysis can be anticipated. Nevertheless, results of simulations and rapidly growing clinical experience indicate that the toxic-to-therapeutic ratio of t-PA is remarkably low. Computer-assisted simulation appears likely to be of value for prospective evaluation and comparison of specific thrombolytic agents and combinations that offer promise, as well as for facilitating development of safe and effective dose regimens tailored to specific clinical applications.

REFERENCES

1. Sobel BE, Gross RW, Robison AK: Thrombolysis, clot selectivity, and kinetics. Circulation 70:160, 1984.
2. Tiefenbrunn AJ, Graor RA, Robison AK, Lucas FV, Hotchkiss A, Sobel BE: Pharmacodynamics of tissue-type plasminogen activator characterized by computer-assisted simulation. Circulation 73:1291, 1986.
3. Tiefenbrunn AJ, Sobel BE: Tissue-type plasminogen activator (t-PA): An agent with promise for selective thrombolysis. Int Cardiol 7:82, 1985.
4. Tiefenbrunn AJ, Robison AK, Kurnik PB, Ludbrook PA, Sobel BE: Clinical pharmacology in patients with evolving myocardial infarction of tissue-type plas-

minogen activator produced by recombinant DNA technology. Circulation 71: 110, 1985.

5. Barshop BA, Wrenn RF, Frieden C: Analysis of numerical methods for computer simulation of kinetic processes: Development of KINSIM—a flexible, portable system. Anal Biochem 130:134, 1983.

6. Graor RA, Risius B, Young JR, Lucas FV, Ruschhaupt WF, Beven EG, Grossbard E: Peripheral artery and bypass graft thrombolysis with recombinant human tissue-type plasminogen activator. Circulation 72(suppl III)(abstr):III-15, 1985.

7. Collen D, Topol EJ, Tiefenbrunn AJ, Gold HK, Weisfeldt ML, Sobel BE, Leinbach RC, Brinker JA, Ludbrook PA, Yasuda I, Bulkley BH, Robison AK, Hutter AM, Bell WR, Spadaro JJ, Khaw BA, Grossbard E: Coronary thrombolysis with recombinant human tissue-type plasminogen activator: A prospective, randomized, placebo-controlled trial. Circulation 7:1012, 1984.

8. Collen D, Bounameaux H, DeCock F, Lijnen HR, Verstraete M: Analysis of coagulation and fibrinolysis during intravenous infusion of recombinant human tissue-type plasminogen activator in patients with acute myocardial infarction. Circulation 73:511, 1986.

9. Williams DO, Borer J, Braunwald E, Chesebro JH, Cohen LS, Dalen J, Dodge HT, Francis CK, Knatterud G, Ludbrook PA, Markis JE, Mueller H, Desvigne-Nickens P, Passamani ER, Powers ER, Rao AK, Roberts R, Ross A, Ryan TJ, Sobel BE, Winniford M, Zaret B, and coinvestigators: Intravenous recombinant tissue-type plasminogen activator in patients with acute myocardial infarction: A report from the NHLBI Thrombolysis in Myocardial Infarction Trial. Circulation 73:338, 1986.

3

Pharmacokinetics of Tissue Plasminogen Activator

Robert A. Baughman, Jr.
Genentech, Inc.
South San Francisco, California

I. INTRODUCTION

The identification of tissue plasminogen activator was made in the 1940s (1,2), but it was not until the isolation of plasminogen activator from human uterine tissue (3) and subsequently its purification and characterization from a melanoma cell line (4) that sufficient quantities could be obtained for thorough study. The activator from the Bowes melanoma cell culture was initially called extrinsic plasminogen activator (EPA), as it represented an activator from the extrinsic pathway. This activator was later identified as tissue-type plasminogen activator (t-PA) and was shown to bind fibrin and effectively activate fibrin-bound plasminogen, converting it to plasmin (5).

Initial production of rt-PA was by a small-scale methodology (Genentech Process Code G11021). This mammalian tissue culture rt-PA (Acti-vase®, Genentech, Inc.) and the melanoma-derived t-PA (mt-PA) were shown to be indistinguishable when the kinetics of plasminogen activation in the presence and absence of fibrin and the disappearance of radioactivity following the bolus administration of ^{125}I-labeled mt-PA and rt-PA were compared (6).

Pharmacokinetic comparison has been demonstrated to be an excellent predictor of thrombolytic differences between t-PAs derived from various sources, and the pharmacokinetic profile has become an integral part of t-PA characterization. This chapter will summarize the t-PA pharmacokinetic literature, focusing on studies with recombinant t-PA (rt-PA).

II. PHARMACOKINETIC STUDIES WITH mt-PA

The euglobulin fibrinolytic activity (EFA) in the plasma of animals and a few human patients provided the first t-PA pharmacokinetic data. Korninger et al. (7) reported that in rabbits receiving bolus mt-PA the EFA declined with a half-life of 2–3 min. The half-life in rabbits of ^{125}I-radioactivity following ^{125}I-mt-PA dosing was similar to the EFA half-life (i.e., 2–5 min) over the first 20 min. This suggested that over this interval the ^{125}I measured in plasma was associated with intact t-PA. Up to 50% of the administered ^{125}I was found in the liver at 20 min. When mt-PA was administered to hepatectomized rabbits (n = 2), there was no significant disappearance of plasma radioactivity within 45 min of dosing (7), indicating that the initial clearance of t-PA is via the hepatic route.

The half-life of fibrinolytic activity, as measured on fibrin plates, after a bolus mt-PA injection in intact, partially, and totally hepatectomized rabbits was 2, 8, and 40 min, respectively (8). In these studies by Nilsson and co-workers, the disposition of ^{125}I following ^{125}I-mt-PA dosing in normal rabbits was described by a three-compartment model. The initial $t_{1/2}$ coincided with the disappearance of the fibrinolytic activity in intact animals (above) and probably reflects t-PA uptake by the eliminating organ(s) (e.g., liver). The half-life of the second compartment was 14 min, which was thought to be related to ^{125}I-mt-PA elimination as well as formation and elimination of inhibitor complexes. The third phase ($t_{1/2}$ approximately 2 hr) reflected a complex function incorporating elimination, the formation of complexes and metabolites, and the generation of free ^{125}I (8).

The organ distribution of ^{125}I in rats injected with 20 ng ^{125}I-mt-PA was determined at 0.05, 0.25, 1, 6, and 72 hr (3, 15, 60, 360, and 4320 min) after dosing. There was an initial, rapid accumulation of ^{125}I-label in the liver (58%), which rapidly decreased to only 5% of the dose after 60 min. These data were qualitatively supported by whole-body autoradiography (8).

Fuchs et al. (9) administered ^{125}I-mt-PA as an i.v. bolus to mice. The total ^{125}I-activity in the plasma was identical to the radioactivity in the precipitate of plasma treated with tricholoracetic acid (TCA), demonstrating that ^{125}I-activity in the first 15 min probably reflects parent compound. The activity in the TCA precipitable material followed multicompartment kinetics. The clearance of ^{125}I-mt-PA was unchanged when administered in the presence of 3 mg macroalbumin, a nonspecific reticuloendothelial system blocking agent. When ^{125}I-mt-PA was administered with 1 mg asialoorosomucoid, the clearance was also unaffected, suggesting that the rapid removal of t-PA from the circulation is not mediated by asialoglycoprotein receptors. In the presence of 1000-fold excess of unlabeled mt-PA, the clearance of ^{125}I-mt-PA was unaltered. This would indicate that the t-PA clearance is nonsaturable or saturable only at high doses. One pathway for rapid, nonsaturable clearance is via glomercular filtration. The clearance of mt-PA was unchanged by functional bilateral nephrectomy, which demonstrates that renal mechanisms are not involved in the rapid clearance of parent mt-PA from the circulation (9).

III. PHARMACOKINETICS OF ONE- AND TWO-CHAIN FORMS OF t-PA

In the course of the purification and characterization of t-PA from the culture fluid of the Bowes melanoma cell line (4), the presence of one- and two-chain (C1 and C2) forms of the t-PA molecule were identified by SDS polyacrylamide gel electrophoresis. However, when human blood vessel perfusate (10) and porcine heart and human uterus (3,11) were extracted in the presence of the protease inhibitor aprotinin, conflicting results were reported.

In rabbits, the half-lives of the euglobulin fibrinolytic activity following C1 and C2 mt-PA dosing were comparable (3 and 2 min, respectively; n = 2). The ^{125}I organ distribution for ^{125}I-labeled C1 and C2 mt-PA was also very similar (7).

In rabbits injected with mt-PA and rt-PA, as either one- or two-chain forms, the initial half-lives were all in the range of 2–3 min (12). When C2 rt-PA was infused in dogs, baboons, and humans, the initial half-lives following cessation of the infusion were 4, 6, and 6 min respectively. Very similar half-lives were obtained in human patients following C2 rt-PA dosing of 0.5 or 0.75 mg/kg. These data in higher animals and man further indicate similar kinetic properties of mt-PA and rt-PA in either the one- or the two-chain form (12).

IV. NONCLINICAL PHARMACOKINETICS OF RECOMBINANT-DERIVED t-PA

Recombinant t-PA was initially produced at Genentech by a small-scale process (Genentech Process Code G11021), and then scaled up to a more commercially efficient process (Genentech Process Codes G11035, G11044). The percentage of one-chain material obtained by the two methods was 1–5 and 70–80%, respectively. Unfortunately, G11021 rt-PA has been referred to as two-chain rt-PA and G11035 and G11044 rt-PA as one-chain material, rather than indicating that they are derived from different processes with different ratios of one- and two-chain product.

The pharmacokinetics and fibrinolytic activity of rt-PA from the two processes have been well characterized. Collen et al. (13) observed that the half-life of plasma disappearance in rabbits for the G11021 material was 2.0 ± 0.1 min as compared to 1.6 ± 1.1 min for the G11035 product. This suggested a slightly slower clearance rate for G11021 rt-PA. A slower plasma clearance for G11021 was given additional support when it was shown that when G11021 and G11035 rt-PA were infused at the same rate into dogs and rabbits, the t-PA plasma concentrations were higher following G11021 administration. In the same study, the fibrinolytic activity in the euglobulin

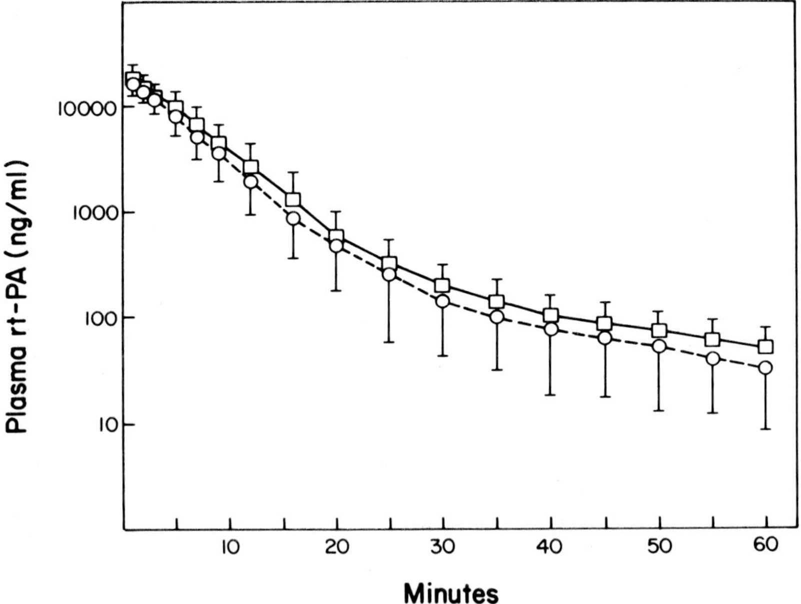

Figure 1   The time course of clearance of C1 rt-PA (○) and C2 rt-PA (□) in rhesus monkeys following 1-mg/kg bolus. Mean ± SD; n = 11 for C1 rt-PA and n = 6 for C2 rt-PA.

fraction decreased more rapidly following infusion of G11035. However, there were no differences observed in thrombolytic properties or fibrin specificity of the two materials (G11021 and G11035) in rabbits with experimental jugular vein thrombosis, or in dogs with coronary artery thrombosis (13).

In attempting to characterize the differences between rt-PA G11021 and G11035, the question focused on the one-chain/two-chain issue, suggesting that the pharmacokinetic difference observed between the material from the two different processes related to "chainedness." To explore this question, rt-PA (G11035, 79.5% one-chain) was subjected to limited plasmin proteolysis which generated two-chain rt-PA (>95% two-chain). The C1 and C2 rt-PA was administered as an intravenous bolus to adult rhesus monkeys. Seventeen blood samples were collected over 60 min. Plasma concentrations (Figure 1) and pharmacokinetic parameter estimates (Table 1) were not statistically different. The differences previously observed between rt-PA G11021 (95% two-chain) and rt-PA G11035 were not observed when the two-chain rt-PA was derived from the one-chain material. The difference in rt-PA biodisposition would appear to be due to some factor other than "chainedness."

V. CLINICAL PHARMACOKINETICS OF TISSUE-TYPE PLASMINOGEN ACTIVATOR

From the first report of therapeutic use of t-PA in man (14), Matsuo estimated the elimination rate constant, half-life, and clearance using an oversimplified one-compartment model and limited plasma concentration-time data (15). The values of $t_{1/2}$ = 2.4 min and CL = 847 ml/min may have provided the first rough pharmacokinetic parameter estimates for t-PA, but should be discarded in light of more complete studies using sensitive and specific analytical procedures. Tiefenbrunn et al., in a study of 12 patients treated for coronary thrombosis, stated that disappearance curves were monoexponential for at least two half-lives (16).

In 1985, Verstraete et al. (17) reported on the pharmacokinetics of rt-PA G11021 in three groups of human patients receiving three different infusion rates (5.6, 8.3, and 10 µg/kg/min). These authors were the first to show in human subjects the multicompartment disposition of rt-PA. Although blood sampling "was not prolonged enough to allow accurate determination of the second exponential term in the plasma disappearance curve" of the three patient groups, a group of healthy volunteers provided estimates of $t_{1/2}$ alpha = 5.2 min and $t_{1/2}$ beta = 55 min. Clearance estimates for all groups ranged from 420 to 800 ml/min. An initial half-life ($t_{1/2}$ alpha) estimate of 5.5 min from four patients studied previously with mt-PA was also reported, which

Table 1   Pharmacokinetic Parameter Estimates for Rhesus Monkeys Receiving Either One- ($>70\%$) or Two-Chain ($>95\%$) rt-PA as a 1-mg/kg i.v. Bolus

	A (ng/ml)	B (ng/ml)	Alpha (min^{-1})	Beta (min^{-1})	$t_{1/2}$Alpha (min)	$t_{1/2}$Beta (min)	$AUC_\circ^\infty$ (μg · min/ml)	V_1 (ml/kg)
One-chain rt-PA (n = 11)								
Mean	22780	392	0.252	0.034	2.75	20.4	107.0	134
± SD	4580	447	0.086	0.012	0.93	7.2	27.6	25
Two-chain rt-PA (n = 6)								
Mean	23970	346	0.207	0.029	3.34	23.9	133.0	126
± SD	5050	174	0.035	0.010	0.56	4.0	42.6	20

No statistically significant differences by unpaired t-test; $p < 0.05$.

agreed with the $t_{1/2}$ alpha estimate for patients and healthy volunteers dosed with rt-PA. Apparent from this work was the large contribution of the initial, alpha phase to the overall disposition.

Garabedian et al. (18) also studied the pharmacokinetics of rt-PA G11021. Four groups of patients (n = 27) with myocardial infarction were studied at infusion rates of 4, 5, 5.5, and 7 µg/kg/min over 90 min, with 10% of the total dose administered initially as a bolus. A fifth group (n = 16) received 8.3 µg/kg/min for 60 min without a loading dose. The five infusion rates resulted in plateau plasma concentrations of 0.52 to 1.4 µg/ml. Although the intersubject variability was substantial, a linear relationship between the plateau concentration and infusion rate was observed (p < 0.001). The disposition kinetics were described by a biexponential (two-compartment) model, with mean initial and terminal half-lives of 5.3 and 46 min for all patients studied (18). As in the previous study (17), the dominance of the alpha phase was observed, as 90% of plateau rt-PA plasma concentrations were achieved in just over four initial phase half-lives. The volume of the central compartment was estimated in those subjects receiving the bolus loading dose to be 7.3 L. This value may be artifactually elevated since it was calculated from the 0.5-min sample rather than the hypothetical concentration at zero time.

The pharmacokinetics of rt-PA G11021 (n = 12) and rt-PA G11035 (n = 6) were compared in patients with myocardial infarction (19). All patients received an intravenous bolus of 10% of the calculated total dose followed by a 90-min constant rate infusion of 4, 5.3, and 7 µg/kg/min in the group receiving rt-PA G11021, and 7, 9.4, and 11 µg/kg/min in the rt-PA G11035 group. Substantial variations in plateau plasma concentrations were apparent. However, infusion of rt-PA G11035 resulted in plateau concentrations approximately 30–35% lower than with comparable infusion rates of rt-PA G11021. Biexponential analysis of the data indicated alpha and beta half-lives for rt-PA G11021 of 5.2 and 46.2 min, as compared to 4.3 and 36.5 min in patients receiving rt-PA G11035. Plasma clearance rates were also greater in those patients receiving rt-PA G11035 (732 ml/min versus 555 ml/min). The volume of the central compartment was comparable between the two groups. These (unreported) data are in excellent agreement with what has been observed in rhesus monkeys.

The pharmacokinetics of rt-PA G11035 was further characterized in eight patients with vascular thromboocclusive disease (20). The patients received 0.25 mg/kg as a 10-min infusion (25 µg/kg/min) with blood samples taken for 70 min following the initiation of the infusion. Plasma concentration data were analyzed by a nonlinear regression procedure utilizing a two-compartment model, and by standard noncompartment procedures (21). The mean parameters generated from these analyses are found in Table 2. Clearance (CL) is the single most important parameter to know when establishing steady-state concentrations (C_{ss}) of a therapeutic agent (22) because steady-state is achieved when the rate of drug entering the body equals the rate of removal. If the desired C_{ss} is known, then the CL will determine the dosing rate. A high degree of confidence is placed in the CL value reported here (550 ml/min) since the same value was calculated using either the specific compartment model or by noncompartmental methods.

The mean pharmacokinetic data from this dosing scheme were used to predict the steady-state rt-PA concentrations in an additional patient who received 0.5 mg/kg over 60 min (8.3 µg/kg/min). This rate falls within the range of dosing rates used in treatment of myocardial infarction. As can be seen in Figure 2, there was excellent agreement between the predicted and actual infusion concentrations. This additional analysis would indicate linear rt-PA pharmacokinetics over the limited range of these clinical dosing regimens. Further, the data would suggest that using kinetic parameters specific to a patient group steady-state rt-PA plasma concentrations may be predicted for a variety of dosage regimens.

The largest rt-PA pharmacokinetic trial was conducted in normal, male volunteers (n = 27) to study three different rt-PA preparations (23). Three groups of nine subjects each received 0.25 mg/kg as a 10-min constant rate infusion. Plasma rt-PA concentrations were measured by an enzyme-linked

Table 2   Pharmacokinetic Parameter Estimates Following a 0.25-mg/kg rt-PA Infusion over 10 Minutes in Eight Patients with Thromboocclusive Disease

	Mean	± SD	Range
Two-compartment model			
$t_{1/2}$ Alpha (min)	4.36	0.94	3.37–5.77
$t_{1/2}$ Beta (min)	26.5	11.0	15.0–47.5
V_1 (L)	3.82	1.40	1.69–6.11
AUC (ng · min/L)	36.3	11.9	21.0–55.8
CL (ml/min)	549	180	269–926
Compartment-independent			
AUC (ng · min/L)	34.3	8.98	23.2–49.3
VD_{ss} (L)	10.3	3.05	5.36–15.1
CL (ml/min)	554	175	304–861

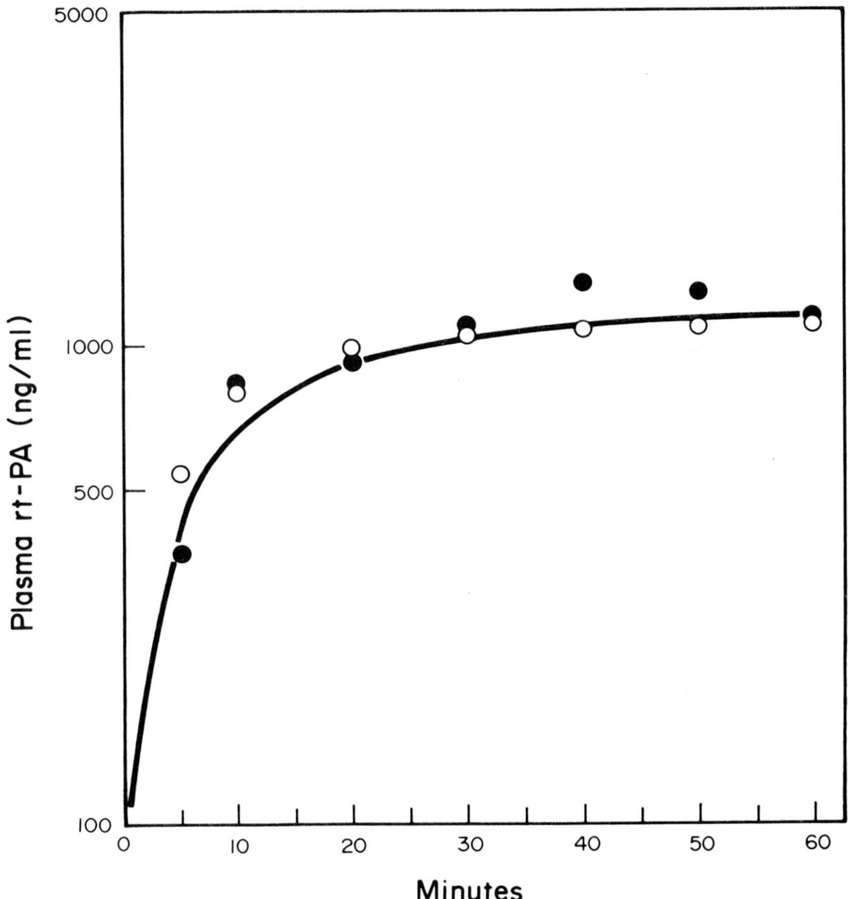

Figure 2   Patient 5 (0.5 mg/kg over 60 min). Predicted (O) and actual (●) plasma concentrations (ng/ml). ___ = Fitted line to actual concentrations.

immunosorbent assay (ELISA), and the data were then fit to a two-compartment model by an iterative, nonlinear regression procedure. The data were also analyzed by noncompartmental methods (e.g., AUC, Vd_{ss}, CL) (21). Mean pharmacokinetic parameter estimates are found in Table 3.

There was no statistically significant difference between groups for any parameter. More important, the pharmacokinetic parameters from young, normal subjects would appear to correlate with data obtained from the older

                                                                BAUGHMAN

Table 3   Comparative Pharmacokinetics of Three Preparations of rt-PA in Normal, Adult Male Human Subjects

		Group 1 (n = 9)	Group 2 (n = 9)	Group 3 (n = 9)
$t_{1/2}$ Alpha (min)	Mean	4.16	3.93	3.60
	SD	1.01	0.69	1.38
$t_{1/2}$ Beta (min)	Mean	30.1	36.0	28.9
	SD	12.0	15.7	14.9
V_1 (L)	Mean	4.31	4.33	4.25
	SD	0.92	1.11	1.48
AUC (ng · min/L)	Mean	28.8	26.7	27.1
	SD	5.10	4.81	5.35
Vd_{ss} (L)	Mean	9.28	12.04	10.95
	SD	2.40	7.13	4.21
CL (ml/min)	Mean	630	730	690
	SD	140	150	140

No statistically significant differences by one-way ANOVA; $p < 0.05$.

patient population. Although $t_{1/2}$ alpha and $t_{1/2}$ beta agree across populations, younger, normal subjects would appear to have an increased clearance. This finding is consistent with established data indicating clearance changes in patients (22).

VI. RECENT BRIEF REPORTS

Three recently published abstracts indicate new areas of rt-PA pharmacokinetic investigation. The first of these reports on the use of isolated, perfused rat liver preparations to examine rt-PA disposition and metabolism at three different perfusion concentrations (0.01, 0.1, and 1 µg/ml) (24). Bile and liver perfusate samples were analyzed for rt-PA following single-pass perfusion of the liver. No rt-PA appeared in the bile. However, a decrease in the percentage of rt-PA extracted by the liver was reported at the highest rt-PA perfusate concentration. Although indicating that rt-PA extraction in this system is saturable at concentrations within the range of those observed clinically, the authors unfortunately extrapolated these results to the clinical setting. Data are available at Genentech showing that clinical plasma rt-PA concentrations could be predicted from averaged parameters determined at a threefold higher dose (resulting in concentrations in excess of 2.5 μg/ml), which would not support the extrapolation of perfused liver data to therapeutics. Considerable work will be needed to determine if rt-PA clearance is saturable within the range of dosage regimens used in treating patients.

The two-compartment model appears at this time to adequately describe rt-PA disposition, mainly due to the large contribution of the initial, alpha phase (>80%) to the total area under the curve. However, more elaborate models based on more extensive data sets in larger study populations will most likely be reported. Seifried et al. (25) have reported using a triexponential model to evaluate data from eighteen subjects receiving 0.25 mg/kg over 10 min.

In extensive work in rodents, Tanswell et al. (26) have reported the use of a three-compartment model with a shorter initial half-life, a second $t_{1/2}$ of approximately 10 min, and a terminal half-life comparable to or slightly longer than the $t_{1/2}$ beta values that have been reported to date. A more complete and detailed pharmacokinetic picture will undoubtedly emerge as the sensitivity and specificity of rt-PA analytical methods is increased, and as more studies with extensive blood sampling schedules are conducted in appropriate animal models and in patients and normal subjects.

REFERENCES

1. Christensen LR, MacLeod CM: Proteolytic enzyme of serum: characterization, activation, and reaction with inhibitors. J Gen Physiol 28:559–583, 1945.
2. Astrup T, Permin PM: Fibrinolysis in animal organism. Nature 159:681–682, 1947.
3. Rijken DC, Wijngaards G, Zaal-DeJong M, Welbergen J: Purification and partial characterization of plasminogen activator from human uterine tissue. Biochim Biophys Acta 580:140, 1979.
4. Rijken DC, Collen D: Purification and characterization of the plasminogen activator secreted by human melanoma cells in culture. J Biol Chem 256:7035–7041, 1981.
5. Hoylaerts M, Rijken DC, Lijnen HR, Collen D: Kinetics of the activation of plasminogen by human tissue plasminogen activator. J Biol Chem 257:2912–2919, 1982.
6. Collen D, Stassen JM, Marafino BJ, Builder S, DeCock F, Ogez J, Tajiri D, Pennica D, Bennett WF, Salwa J, Hoyng CF: Biological properties of human tissue-type plasminogen activator obtained by expression of recombinant DNA in mammalian cells. J Pharmacol Exp Ther 231:146–152, 1984.

7. Korninger C, Stassen JM, Collen D: Turnover of human extrinsic (tissue-type) plasminogen activator in rabbits. Thromb Haemostas 46:658–661, 1981.

8. Nilsson S, Einarsson M, Ekvarn S, Haggroth L, Mattsson Ch: Turnover of tissue plasminogen activator in normal and hepatectomized rabbits. Thromb Res 39: 511–521, 1985.

9. Fuchs HE, Berger H Jr, Pizzo SV: Catabolism of human tissue plasminogen activator in mice. Blood 65:539–544, 1985.

10. Binder BR, Spragg J, Austen KF: Purification and characterization of human vascular plasminogen activator derived from blood vessel perfusates. J Biol Chem 254:1998–2003, 1979.

11. Wallen P, Ranby M, Bergsdorf N, Kok P: Purification and characterization of tissue plasminogen activator: on the occurrence of two different forms and their enzymatic properties. In *Progress in Fibrinolysis,* vol. 5, Davidson JP, Nilsson IM, Astedt B, Eds., Churchill Livingstone, Edinburgh, 1981, pp. 16–23.

12. Bounameaux H, Verstraete M, Collen D: Comparative pharmacokinetics of human tissue-type plasminogen activator (tPA) obtained from cell culture (Bowes melanoma) or by recombinant DNA technology. Thromb Haemostas 54:61, 1985.

13. Collen D, Lijnen HR, Van der Werf F, Hotchkiss A, Lubinecki AS, Builder SE, Hoyng CF: Biological and thrombolytic properties of one-chain and two-chain forms of human tissue-type plasminogen activator (t-PA) obtained by expression of recombinant DNA in mammalian cells (in press).

14. Weimar W, Stibbe J, van Seyen AJ, Billiau A, DeSomer P, Collen D: Specific lysis of an iliofemoral thrombus by administration of extrinsic (tissue-type) plasminogen activator. Lancet 2:1018–1020, 1981.

15. Matsuo O: Turnover of tissue plasminogen activator in man. Thromb Haemostas 48:242, 1982.

16. Tiefenbrunn AJ, Robison AK, Kurneck PB, Ludbrook PA, Sobel BE: Clinical pharmacology in patients with evolving myocardial infarction of tissue-type plasminogen activator produced by recombinant DNA technology. Circulation 71:110–116, 1985.

17. Verstraete M, Bounameaux H, deCock F, Van der Werf F, Collen D: Pharmacokinetics and systemic fibrinolytic effects of recombinant human tissue-type plasminogen activator (rt-PA) in humans. J Pharmacol Exp Ther 235:506–512, 1985.

18. Garabedian HD, Gold HK, Leinbach RC, Yasuda T, Johns JA, Collen D: Dose-dependent thrombolysis, pharmacokinetics and hemostatic effects of recombinant human tissue-type plasminogen activator for coronary thrombolysis. Amer J Cardiol 58:673–679, 1986.

19. Garabedian HD, Gold HK, Leinbach RC, Johns JA, Yasuda T, Kanke M, Collen D: Comparative properties of two clinical preparations of recombinant human tissue-type plasminogen activator in patients with acute myocardial infarction. JACC (in press).

20. Grossbard EB, Baughman RA, Benninger AH: Clinical pharmacokinetics of recombinant human tissue-type plasminogen activator produced in suspension

culture (rt-PA [Code G11035]) in patients with thrombo-occlusive disease. Data on file, Genentech, Inc., South San Francisco, California, 1986.

21. Gibaldi M, Perrier D: *Pharmacokinetics,* 2nd ed,, Marcel Dekker, New York, 1982, pp. 409–416.

22. Benet LZ, Sheiner LB: Pharmacokinetics: The dynamics of drug absorption, distribution and elimination, and Design and optimization of dosage regimens: pharmacokinetic data. In *Goodman and Gilman's The Pharmacological Basis of Therapeutics,* 7th ed., Gilman AG, Goodman LS, Rall TW, Murad F, Eds., Macmillan, New York, 1985.

23. Grossbard E, Baughman RA: Comparative pharmacokinetics of three preparations of recombinant human tissue-type plasminogen activator (rt-PA) produced in suspension culture. Data on file, Genentech, Inc., South San Francisco, California, 1986.

24. Fong K-L, Lynn RK: Disposition and metabolism of tissue-type plasminogen activator (tPA) in the isolated perfused rat liver. The Pharmacologist 28:117, 1986.

25. Siefried E, Tanswell P, Su CAPF, Feuerer W, Pindur G, Heimpel H: Recombinant tissue-type plasminogen activator (rt-PA): pharmacokinetics and effects on coagulation and fibrinolytic system in healthy volunteers. In *Fibrinolysis,* Abstracts of the 8th Int. Cong. on Fibrinolysis, Vienna, A242, 1986.

26. Tanswell P, Busch U, Zipp H: Whole body autoradiography and pharmacokinetics of recombinant tissue-type plasminogen activator (rt-PA) in the rat. In *Fibrinolysis,* Abstracts of the 8th Int. Cong. on Fibrinolysis, Vienna, A221, 1986.

MYOCARDIAL INFARCTION

4

Thrombolysis in Acute Myocardial Infarction

H. J. C. Swan
Cedars-Sinai Medical Center
Los Angeles, California

William Ganz
University of California at Los Angeles
School of Medicine
and Cedars-Sinai Medical Center
Los Angeles, California

The clinical syndrome of acute myocardial infarction is caused by limitation of coronary blood flow of a magnitude and duration so as to result in necrosis of a significant quantity of myocardium. The purpose of this chapter is to outline the role of thrombus in producing complete coronary occlusion and intense myocardial ischemia, and the experience with thrombolytic agents other than tissue-type plasminogen activator (t-PA), which is extensively discussed elsewhere in this monograph. Some of the broader implications for large-scale treatment of myocardial infarction with thrombolytic agents are also considered.

I. PATHOPHYSIOLOGY OF ACUTE MYOCARDIAL INFARCTION

Coronary Artery Disease

The underlying pathological cause of acute myocardial infarction is atherosclerotic coronary artery disease in 99% of subjects. The disease can involve any artery in any location. For practical purposes, however, proximal location and a sizable "territory at risk"—that myocardium supplied by the diseased artery (10–40% myocardial mass)—are involved in patients who present with clinical manifestations of myocardial infarction. The degree of coronary obstruction caused by atherosclerosis alone varies from subtotal in most patients to mild (less than 60% of luminal cross-section area) in a small population of patients. The specific pathology involving the coronary artery itself is complex.

Thrombus usually occurs at the site of a coronary artery stenosis where an atheromatous plaque has ulcerated, probably due to perforation of a cholesterol abscess. The disrupted plaque exposes positively charged subintimal collagen and connective tissue fragments in the coronary wall to the negatively charged circulating platelets. The interaction initiates platelet adhesion, subsequent platelet aggregation, and secondary induction of the clotting cascade to form a fibrin-platelet coronary artery thrombus.

In 10–25% of patients with acute infarction, there is a subtotal—rather than total—coronary artery occlusion that is also due to coronary artery thrombus (1,2). There is ample evidence that unstable angina (3–5) and even sudden coronary death (6) also result from an acute thrombotic complication of a disrupted atheromatous plaque. The underlying pathophysiology in patients with acute infarction is similar for both total and subtotal coronary occlusion. Although patients with subtotal occlusion undergo myocardial necrosis at a slower rate, these patients are at risk of infarct extension and its associated adverse prognosis as a consequence of progression to total coronary occlusion.

Myocardial Necrosis

Myocardial infarction is due to a reduction of coronary blood flow to a region of myocardium for a time interval sufficient to cause its necrosis. The exact mechanism of initiation of necrosis has not been precisely defined. Deprivation of metabolic substrate, incomplete removal of metabolic products, both or other mechanisms—whatever the cause, necrosis commences approximately 20–30 min following complete deprivation of antegrade blood flow at normal body temperature (7) and progresses outward from the subendocardial myocardium to the subepicardial (Figure 1) zones. In general, the rate of progression of myocardial necrosis is inversely related to the magnitude of residual perfusion of the ischemic myocardium and is slower when an infarction is due to subtotal rather than total coronary artery occlusion or when there are well-developed collateral vessels (8,9). The potential influence of collateral flow on the rate of myocardial necrosis is illustrated by species differences in the level of collateral flow immediately after occlusion of the

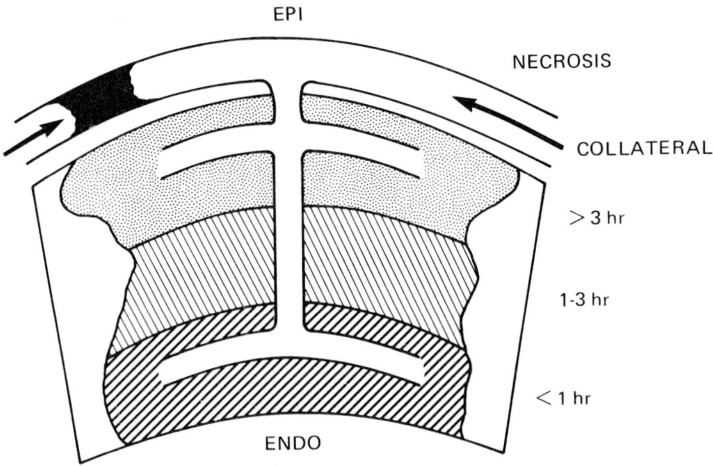

Figure 1   Complete occlusion of a coronary artery supplying a territory of significant magnitude results in effects on that territory. The diagram represents a completely occluded artery (top left coronary flow from left to right). Collateral flow of small magnitude is possible through the remaining coronary bed. There is maximal vasodilation in both the subendocardial and subepicardial intramyocardial vessels. Any residual blood flow via collaterals will be preferentially directed to the subepicardial layers of the myocardium. Thus, subendocardial flow approaches zero, and subepicardial flow may be 5–15% of normal. As a consequence, there is a progressive increase in the proportion of the territory at risk which passes from the ischemic state. An approximate time scale is placed to the right of the figure with maximal myocardial destruction between 1 and 3 hr in the example given.

coronary artery via congenitally present epicardial collateral connections (9). In the rabbit, the sheep, and the pig there is virtually no coronary collateral circulation and consequently myocardial necrosis progresses rapidly and is usually complete within 58 min after coronary occlusion, whereas in the guinea pig there is no myocardial necrosis following coronary artery occlusion, possibly due to extensive and well-developed congenital collateral vessels. Studies of myocardial perfusion and studies of myocardial viability and function (10,11) suggest that the pattern and time sequence of myocardial necrosis following complete occlusion of the coronary artery in man may be similar to that in dogs and monkeys, and myocardial necrosis is generally complete within about 4 hr of total and persistent occlusion. Significant myocardial salvage can sometimes be achieved following longer periods of ischemia in patients in whom the artery of infarction is not totally or persistently occluded or in whom there are well-developed collateral vessels present prior to infarction (Figure 2).

Hemodynamic factors may also influence the rate of myocardial necrosis. Both hypotension and tachycardia can further decrease perfusion to the acutely ischemic myocardium and thereby accelerate the rate of necrosis and

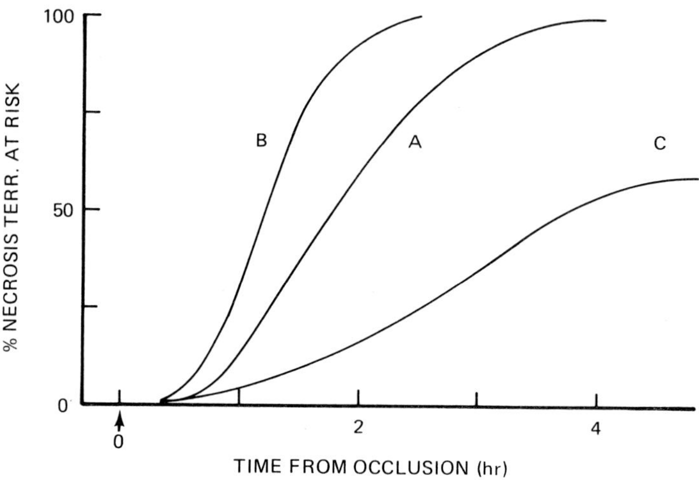

Figure 2   Increase in the proportion of myocardium in the territory at risk passing to the necrotic state as a function of time. From the onset of complete coronary occlusion and in the absence of substantive collateral flow, necrosis commences at 20–30 min and progresses to completion in 3–5 hr. The steepest part of the slope (defining the time of maximal loss of ischemic but still viable tissue) probably lies at approximately 2 hr. Curve B represents a "worst case" situation. This postulates an individual with relatively mild (50±% stenosis) coronary artery disease. If such an individual develops an acute thrombus and the territory at risk is large, the patient might be expected to suffer acute cardiac collapse, potentially fatal arrhythmias, and, in the absence of preformed collaterals and an adequate perfusion pressure, could potentially develop complete transmural necrosis in 1–2 hr. The more favorable curve C represents an individual with preexisting significant coronary disease, continued myocardial ischemia, predeveloped collateral vessels, and a hypertensive response to the acute event. In this situation, the preservation of the middle and subepicardial layers of myocardium may be quite prolonged. Occasionally a substantive proportion of myocardium remains viable, and indeed functional, perfused by collateral vessels alone.

reduce the potential for myocardial salvage. These hemodynamic factors may be especially important in patients with multiple-vessel coronary artery disease, in whom the arteries supplying the collaterals may have significant proximal stenoses, and therefore relatively small falls in systemic blood pressure may significantly reduce collateral perfusion pressure.

The Dynamic Nature of Acute Myocardial Infarction

The clinical consequences of coronary artery occlusion cannot be considered under a single pathophysiological heading. In acute myocardial infarction it is essential to define at least four pathophysiological phases (12) to roughly encompass those elements of the illness that are fundamentally different from one another in their nature and require separate consideration and therapy:

1. Ischemia—the myocardium in the territory of risk is noncontractile and probably less compliant, has not yet proceeded to necrosis, and will ultimately regain function if blood flow is restored.
2. Necrosis—all of the myocardium in the territory at risk that is destined to undergo necrosis has become necrotic.
3. Compensation—associated with thinning and absorption of the necrotic myocardium and increased activity of the neurohumoral compensatory mechanisms.
4. Healing—dominated by the formation and maturation of scar tissue and limitation of the adverse mechanical consequences of the infarction per se.

Clearly, these pathological subsets overlap considerably.

Of critical importance to the topic of this chapter—coronary reperfusion—is the phase of ischemia (Phase 1). It is convenient to develop a subset within this phase, during which an increasing proportion of myocardium in the territory at risk is passing from the state of ischemia into the state of necrosis (Phase 1a—mixed pathology) (Table 1). From the definitions above, it is obvious that *thrombolytic therapy can only be of value in the phase of ischemia or mixed pathology.* As the proportion of necrotic myocardium within the territory at risk increases, the potential long-term benefit of this intervention declines proportionately. Reestablishment of perfusion in the territory at risk is useful only when a significant mass of jeopardized but still viable myocardium is present. Interventions designed to result in revascularization after the phases of ischemia and mixed pathology are complete can have no influence on the preservation of ischemic and jeopardized myocar-

Table 1   Temporal Phases in the Genesis of Acute Myocardial Infarction

Phase		Pathology	Duration[a]
1.	Ischemia	Reversible normal	20–60 min
1a.	Mixed		
2.	Necrosis	Completed infarct	60 min–5 hr
3.	Compensation	Absorption-thinning-fibrosis	12 hr–2 wk
4.	Healing	Scar formation and contraction	1–6 mo

[a]The ranges vary widely.

dium. While beneficial effects can apparently be demonstrated occasionally from late interventions, they must be associated with mechanisms other than preservation of ischemic myocardium in the initial territory at risk. Prudence would also suggest that restoration of blood flow into completely necrotic myocardium is unlikely to be beneficial and is potentially harmful. The myocardium salvaged by reperfusion gradually recovers in structure and function (13,14–16), whereas irreversibly damaged myocardium undergoes accelerated contraction band necrosis, swelling, and absorption of calcium (13, 15–20). Intramyocardial hemorrhage may occur in regions of advanced necrosis involving not only the myocardium but also the intramyocardial vasculature (14,18,21–24). This "reperfusion hemorrhage" is always confined to the necrotic myocardium (22).

II. OBJECTIVE OF THROMBOLYSIS

It is evident from the above considerations that thrombolysis is not a comprehensive treatment for an evolving acute myocardial infarction. It addresses only one part of the tissue, albeit an important one, namely the proximate cause of the acute obstruction. That coronary obstruction may occur due to thrombosis, or that other changes may cause further complications, is obvious. As demonstrated 32 years ago by Agress and colleagues (25), the philosophical goal of coronary reperfusion is to reestablish the situation prior to the onset of thrombosis and allow time for a more considered evaluation of the disease without paying the penalty of extensive myocardial damage. A primary objective is to preserve or restore myocardial function, which re-

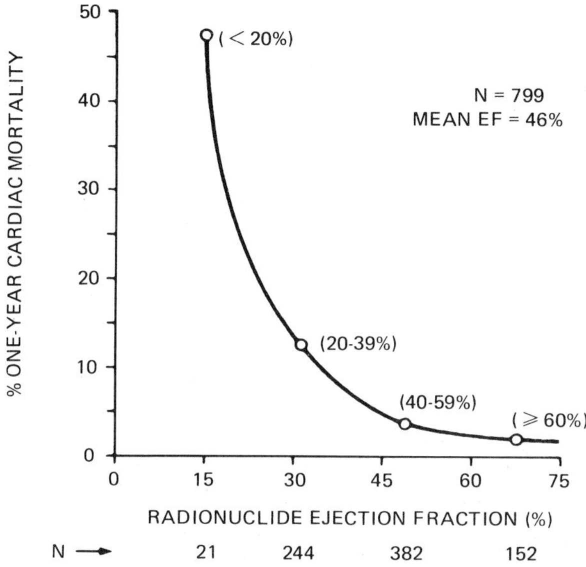

Figure 3   Data of the Multicenter Postinfarction Research Group. Relationship of left ventricular ejection value to survival at 20 months. Of the total of 41,092 patients, the majority had myocardial infarction of moderate magnitude. Of patients whose ejection fraction at rest exceeded 0.5, the 20-month survival exceeded 96%. Of those patients who had an ejection fraction of less than 0.30, the 20-month survival was approximately 70%, and for those with ejection fractions of 0.2 or less, survival was 40–50%. This demonstrates the significance of myocardial destruction in both short- and long-term outcomes of this clinical syndrome. (From Ref. 26.)

mains the single most important determinant of prognosis following myocardial infarction (Figure 3) (26).

Thus, at least four specific elements are relevant to the patient with an acute syndrome leading to myocardial infarction: atherosclerosis, thrombosis, myocardial response, and arrhythmias. It is appropriate to redesignate the objectives of management of acute myocardial infarction as: preservation of life, salvage of the maximum amount of jeopardized myocardium in the territory at risk, stabilization of disorders of cardiac function or cardiac rhythm, and evaluation and management of underlying coronary disease. The latter, important objective is outside the scope of this chapter. Prompt revascularization probably has an effect in all of these objectives.

III. CLINICAL STUDIES ON THROMBOLYSIS

Studies using t-PA are discussed extensively elsewhere in this monograph.

In spite of prior experiences with pharmacological thrombolysis (intravenous) in the 1960s and early '70s (27), current interest in nonsurgical reperfusion dates from the single catheterization experience of Rentrop et al. (28) in dispersing a thrombus in a right coronary artery by use of a guidewire, with striking clinical benefits. Direct mechanical dispersion of an intracoronary thrombus with immediate dilation (angioplasty) of the underlying coronary disease has again been recommended as a primary mode of treatment for acute evolving myocardial infarction (29).

Intracoronary Streptokinase

Direct infusion of thrombolytic substances into the acutely obstructed coronary artery has been demonstrated to result in restoration of blood flow (30,31). However, intracoronary administration of thrombolytic agents requires a complex logistical system, including effective transportation, emergency-room services with a ''standby'' catheterization laboratory, and a workable on-call system. Under favorable circumstances, these factors increase the minimal interval from identification to initiation of effective thrombolytic therapy by 1 to 1½ hr. In addition, maintenance of these logistical arrangements and application of intracoronary reperfusion are restricted to hospitals with effective catheterization laboratories—less than 10% of community hospital facilities.

Intravenous Streptokinase

Early administration of relatively large doses of thrombolytic agents (streptokinase) intravenously has been employed extensively and widely (32,33). This approach had significant advantages over the intracoronary administration, including a reduction in the delay from the onset of coronary occlusion to application of therapy in an emergency room, a wider application of early reperfusion to institutions and physicians without immediate access to catheterization facilities, the potential of reducing the interval even further by application of therapy in a transportation vehicle or at home, and a possible reduction in overall cost. Also, the occluding thrombus appears to become progressively more resistant with time to thrombolytic agents, possibly because of maturation and also by extension distally down the obstructed vessel. A lower blood concentration of thrombolytic agent is achieved intravenously in comparison to local concentration during intracoronary administration; thus, a larger total dose must be faster. Bleeding complications may be expected to be more frequent in intravenous administration than in intracoronary administration.

Results of Thrombolytic Therapy

Information as to efficacy of thrombolytic therapy may be drawn from several sources: the intracoronary and the intravenous studies classified as experiential (observational) reports and the more formal randomized trials. Intravenous followed by intracoronary administration of lytic agents has been reported (34). All these studies largely address reestablishment of vessel patency with additional information as to short-term mortality, ventricular function, and complication rates. Many are flawed in regard to the primary hypothesis regarding the "time window" applicable to the majority of patients (see Figure 1). When a fundamental biological principle is defied (for example, in several studies an average of 6 or more hours elapsed from symptom onset to treatment), the demonstration of any positive benefit would be surprising.

Intracoronary Randomized Trials

A number of such studies have now appeared (7,35). In general, the numbers of patients are small. The frequency of opening of such vessels varies from under 50% to over 80%. A higher opening rate is demonstrated in patients with shorter intervals from onset of infarcted myocardium. The incidence of acute reocclusion in such patients is 10–20%. In several studies a reduction in short-term mortality appeared to be achieved, but it was not always of statistical significance. A significant proportion of patients in these reports were referred for prompt coronary bypass surgery, a few for percutaneous transluminal coronary angioplasty.

Intracoronary Experiential Reports

These nonrandomized experiences may reflect a somewhat different patient population and therapeutic approach to the management of acute myocardial infarction (30,31). Close, "hands-on" attendance during the clinical course was the rule. The reported patency rate was acceptable—60 to 85%. Mortality compared to "concurrent controls," or to prior experience, appeared favorable. No specific conclusion can be made on this particular issue since confounding variables clearly exist in many instances. Experiential reports relative to patients presenting in cardiogenic shock indicate that, in some examples in this highest-risk category, prompt restoration of blood flow was associated with greatly increased survival.

Intravenous Randomized Trials

The principal clinical interest today in reperfusion by thrombolytic agents involves intravenous administration as a practical matter (27). The actual status of the coronary arteries, complete versus subtotal occlusion, the vessel of infarction, the magnitude of the territory at risk, and other aspects may not be definable in advance. In several randomized trials, an anatomical knowledge of the vessels prior to treatment was required; hence, the time of intervention was necessarily delayed and the interval from the onset of occlusion to the onset of reperfusion was extended substantively. The incidence of reperfusion in these patients varied from under 40% to greater than 80%. A significant incidence of bleeding complications was reported. Several randomized trials attempted to investigate more than one phenomenon (with a change of protocol during the study). In general, mortality appeared to be reduced in comparison to controls.

Intravenous Experiential Reports

A number of studies claim an apparent efficacy of this treatment form (32, 33,36). Intravenous thrombolytic therapy was commenced at the earliest possible time and usually prior to angiography. Evidence of reperfusion was obtained by indirect (clinical) methods that may lack specificity as to completeness of occlusion. The incidence of subtotal occlusion has been estimated at 20% of patients with myocardial infarction. A significant (10–20%) proportion did not undergo angiography for a variety of reasons. Nevertheless, a reduction in hospital mortality and apparent improvement in a wide series of clinical indices (including chest pain, nitroglycerin requirement, antiarrhythmic therapy, and heart failure medication) are reported.

Koran and colleagues (37) reported on very early intravenous streptokinase treatment in 53 patients. The mean time to the beginning of treatment was 1.7 hr; treatment was started in the home in nine patients. Achieved patency rate in the total study was 81%. Ejection fraction in seven of the nine home-treated patients averaged 0.67, in contrast to 0.48 in 41 of 44 patients treated in the hospital. An unusually low rate of reperfusion with intravenous streptokinase (36%) reported in a single trial (38) may be due to both delay and prior angiography, which may alter the characteristic of the thrombus itself, and thus the efficacy of specific lytic agents.

IV. PROTOCOL

Patients are considered candidates for thrombolytic therapy if they are seen within 3 hr of the onset of persistent pain that is not relieved by nitroglycerin, with ST-segment elevations in at least two adjacent leads and if there is no contraindication to thrombolytic therapy and anticoagulation. If the pain is intermittent the 3-hr time limit does not apply and the patient is admitted as long as he is symptomatic and the ECG shows acute changes. In patients with contraindication to thrombolytic therapy, primary angioplasty is initiated.

If informed consent is obtained, an intravenous bolus of 40 U/kg of heparin is administered, followed by a 20–30-min infusion of 750,000 U of streptokinase. In patients weighing more than 75 kg, a 1.5-million-U infusion of streptokinase is given over 40–60 min. Following streptokinase, an infusion of heparin is begun, initially at 10 U/kg/hr, and later adjusted to keep the PTT between 50 and 60 s. If no intervention is planned, the heparin is gradually replaced with Coumadin. Anticoagulation with Coumadin is maintained for 2 months. The patient must be warned of the potential consequences of stopping anticoagulation. If signs of reperfusion do not appear within 90 min of the initiation of streptokinase infusion, urgent angiography may be considered for reopening the occluded artery by angioplasty.

Patients admitted in cardiogenic shock or heart failure are treated in the emergency room and moved as soon as possible to the catheterization laboratory for angiography and additional intervention if appropriate. Endotracheal intubation should be avoided if at all possible because it can be the source of serious bleeding.

Anticoagulation is not interrupted during angiography or in preparation for coronary bypass surgery.

In case of reocclusion or appearance of postinfarct angina, the treatment with streptokinase is repeated and early angiography performed to determine the need for secondary angioplasty. If reocclusion occurs more than 5 days after the initial treatment, urokinase is used instead of streptokinase.

In patients with prior infarcts, with a prior history of angina pectoris, or in whom a submaximal predischarge stress test shows significant reversible ischemia, an angiography should be performed.

If anticoagulation has to be discontinued, urgent angioplasty should be considered to reduce the probability of coronary artery reocclusion after discontinuation of anticoagulation.

V. RECOGNITION OF REPERFUSION

Angiographic Signs

Angiographic patency is the "gold standard" of successful reperfusion. The first angiographic sign of reperfusion is frequently the establishment of a sluggish flow of contrast through the thrombus. In both experimental and clinical studies, the lumen and coronary flow generally increase as thrombolysis continues, although sometimes a cyclic pattern of reperfusion and reocclusion may occur before definitive reperfusion is achieved. Neither nitroglycerin nor calcium channel blockers have proved effective in relieving this intermittent occlusion.

Nonangiographic Clinical Signs

In many studies using intravenous administration of thrombolytic agents, pretreatment coronary angiography is not performed in order to minimize the delay and in such studies, recognition of coronary artery reperfusion is based on clinical, nonangiographic criteria.

Abatement of Symptoms

The time of reperfusion is signaled by rapid and progressive relief of chest pain. The patient usually also appears well. Occasionally, reperfusion is preceded by a period of fluctuation of chest pain (39) consistent with the intermittency of patency observed angiographically.

Decrease in ST-Segment and T-Wave Amplitude

Reperfusion is followed by rapid resolution ischemic ST-T wave changes, with a more than 50% decrease in ST elevation over 20 min.

Ventricular Arrhythmias

Accelerated idioventricular rhythm (AIVR) occurs at the time of reperfusion or shortly thereafter in about 40–50% of patients, especially when the ischemia was extensive and severe. Ventricular ectopic beats that occur late in diastole, singly, or as ventricular bigeminy or trigeminy and sometimes form fusion beats are also frequently noted at about the time of reperfusion.

Conduction Blocks

When present, atrioventricular block and intraventricular conduction delays often disappear shortly after reperfusion.

Cardiac Enzyme Washout

The release into the circulation of creatine kinase (CK) and the other cardiac enzymes is accelerated by reperfusion. Following cell death and disruption of the cell plasma membrane, intracellular proteins escape into the interstitial myocardial spaces and from there enter the circulation directly. When antegrade coronary blood flow is reestablished, an abrupt and marked acceleration of CK ''washout'' results in an abrupt and marked rise in serum CK activity by more than 15% of the peak activity in the first hour of rise. A peak level is usually reached within 12 hr of reperfusion, whereas in the absence of reperfusion, serum levels of CK usually remain within the normal range of about 6–8 hr after the onset of infarction and peak about 20–25 hr later. Early reperfusion appears to result in a more complete and rapid washout of CK from the myocardium. The peak serum CK activity as well as the total CK release are considerably higher following reperfusion (2–3 times higher in canine models) than for a nonreperfused myocardial infarction of equivalent size. The significance of early CK washout has been a subject of some controversy (40).

We consider the simultaneous relief of chest pain, resolution of ST-segment elevation, and rapid CK washout following thrombolytic therapy to be reliable indicators of coronary artery reperfusion.

VI. EFFECTS ON MORTALITY

Yusuf and colleagues (27) recently overviewed the mortality outcome in the available published randomized controlled trials. Between 1959 and 1984, a total of 24 randomized trials of intravenous fibrinolytic treatment, involving a total of some 6000 patients, were reported. Four of these trials involved intravenous urokinase. There were nine smaller trials of intercoronary streptokinase involving about 1000 patients collectively. Yusuf concluded that an overview of these data (largely collected in the early 1970s) indicated that intravenous streptokinase produced a highly significant reduction (22%) in the likelihood of death (nearly identical to the results of the GISSI trial referred to below).

Similar favorable trends regarding mortality were deduced from the intracoronary randomized studies. Yusuf and colleagues (27) stressed the need for intravenous streptokinase protocols that addressed practical issues, and the requirement that several thousand patients be effectively randomized into a treatment and control group on the basis of a relatively uniform set of conditions. Studies from the Netherlands (41) and Italy [the GISSI trial (42)] provided substantial support for Yusuf's hypothesis.

The GISSI trial (42) recruited 11,806 of 31,826 patients admitted in 176 participating Italian coronary-care units (CCU) over a 17-month interval. Reasons for exclusion included an interval of more than 12 hr from the onset of symptoms (51%), contraindications to streptokinase therapy (20%), and doubtful myocardial infarction (18%). Complete data were available for analysis, in 99% of the 11,806 patients randomized either to control (which did not require modification of the therapeutic practice of the participating CCU) or to the addition of intravenous infusion of 1.5 million U of streptokinase over 1 hr. No significant differences in the characteristics of patients on admission, prognostic factors, or cardiovascular drugs administered in the hospital could be detected. The 14–21-day in-hospital mortality was 10.7% for the treated group versus 13% for the control group, or a favorable relative risk ratio of 0.81. Greatest benefit appeared in those patients treated at <3 hr (relative risk 0.74); beneficial effect appeared to be lost in the patients randomized between 9 and 12 hr. These differences are highly significant. A further analysis of the 1277 patients randomized within 1 hr after the onset of pain indicated that the treated group enjoyed a major reduction in in-hospital mortality of approximately 47%. Groups favorably affected were patients without prior myocardial infarction and less than 65 years of age and those with multiple or anterior infarct locations. The authors concluded that intravenous infusion of 1.5 million U of streptokinase can be recommended as a safe treatment for all patients with no positive contraindications who can be treated within 6 hr of the onset of pain.

VII. COMPLICATIONS ASSOCIATED WITH THROMBOLYSIS

The principal complications of thrombolytic agents are associated with bleeding. Since streptokinase is the commonly used agent, most of the reported complications are concerned with it. t-PA is believed to be less likely to cause such events, although no significant difference between t-PA and streptokinase with respect to bleeding complications have been reported in a randomized trial. The confounding effects of concomitant use of heparin and variation in postprocedural management render the interpretation of exact mechanisms difficult. Bleeding complications have been noted in all reports on thrombolytic therapy. They may be insignificant—skin bruising or localized hematoma—or severe—stroke, gastrointestinal bleeding, or retroperitoneal hematoma. Intraabdominal bleeding, intrapulmonary bleeding, and hematuria, hemopericardium, and hemothorax have all been reported. Allergic reactions to streptokinase, although suspected, appear to be uncommon.

Reocclusion is an important early and late complication of thrombolytic therapy. As stated, thrombolytic therapy is intended only to resolve the acute occlusion and restore perfusion to the myocardium. It does not necessarily affect the stability of the occluding atherosclerotic obstructive disease, although the residual obstruction appears to decrease spontaneously after successful thrombolytic reperfusion. Reocclusion is most common in patients with the most severe degrees of coronary obstructive disease (<90%) or in whom effective anticoagulation is not achieved or in whom anticoagulation is deliberately or inadvertently discontinued.

VIII. TREATMENT OF MYOCARDIAL INFARCTION IN THE THROMBOLYSIS ERA

It now appears to be clear that acute thrombosis is the precipitating cause of acute myocardial infarction and that, under appropriate circumstances, thrombolysis is effective in dissolving the obstructing thrombus with acceptable levels of complications and side effects.

Verstraete concludes that intravenous administration of a thrombolytic agent is the only realistic therapeutic approach in evolving myocardial infarction in the community (43). He also concludes that short and simple therapeutic schemes must be developed. Using relatively conservative assumptions, systemic administration of streptokinase or t-PA would result in a reperfusion rate of at least 80%, possibly applicable to 90% of all patients. This allows a potential overall reperfusion seven times more than the corresponding figure for the intracoronary approach alone. Widely applicable protocols must be based on the intravenous administration of the most effective and safest thrombolytic agent. While streptokinase has been satisfactory, t-PA may be equally or more effective and have fewer or milder side effects.

In addition, application of the acylated derivatives of streptokinase resulted in a reperfusion rate of 89% (angiographically determined) (44). There was, however, bleeding at arterial and venous puncture sites in most patients. The incidence of reocclusion was low. One of these agents, BRL 26921, is now undergoing randomized clinical trials. In all instances, however, the dominance of the "time window" relative to the phases of ischemia or mixed pathology must be, and will remain, the determinant of outcome.

Lysis of an obstructing thrombus in a diseased coronary artery effectively "buys time." In addition, immediate mortality is significantly reduced, in particular, in those patients receiving prompt treatment early in their disease. While the above analyses are of great importance and serve as a strong base for future investigations on the topic, the present and future availability of more effective fibrinolytic agents and the potential of initiating treatment prior to arrival in an emergency room may alter the basic structure of the needed randomized trials.

In summary, the available thrombolytic agents appear to be effective in the early phase of acute myocardial infarction in regard to reestablishment of vessel patency. The potential expanded role of t-PA is discussed elsewhere in this volume. The weight of evidence indicates that early reperfusion is associated with dramatic reduction in early mortality.

REFERENCES

1. DeWood MA, Spores J, Notske R, Mouser LT, Burroughs R, Golden MS, Lang HT: Prevalence of total coronary occlusion during the early hours of transmural myocardial infarction. N Engl J Med 303:897–902, 1981.
2. Stadius ML, Maynard C, Fritz JK, Davis K, Ritchie JL, Sheehan F, Kennedy JW: Coronary anatomy and left ventricular function in the first 12 hours of acute myocardial infarction: the Western Washington Randomized Intracoronary Streptokinase Trial. Circulation 72:292–301, 1985.
3. Vetrovec GW, Cowley MJ, Overton H, Richardson DW: Intracoronary thrombus in syndromes of unstable myocardial ischemia. Am Heart J 102:1202–1208, 1981.
4. Zack PM, Ischinger T, Aker UT, Dincer B, Kennedy HL: The occurrence of angiographically detected intracoronary thrombus in patients with unstable angina pectoris. Am Heart J 108:1408–1412, 1984.
5. Sherman CT, Litvack F, Grundfest W, Lee M, Chaux A, Kass R, Swan HJC, Matloff J, Forrester JS: Fiberoptic coronary angioscopy identifies thrombus in all patients with unstable angina. Circulation 72(III):112, 1985.
6. Davies MJ, Thomas AC: Thrombosis and acute coronary-artery lesions in sudden cardiac ischemic death. N Engl J Med 310:1137–1140, 1984.
7. Rymer KA, Lowe JE, Rasmussen MM, Jennings RB: The wave-front phenomenon of ischemic cell death. I. Myocardial infarct size vs. duration of coronary occlusion in dogs. Circulation 56:786, 1977.
8. Schaper W, Pasyk S: Influence of collateral flow on the ischemic tolerance of the heart following acute and subacute coronary occlusion. Circulation 53(I):I-57–I-62, 1976.
9. Schaper W: *The Collateral Circulation of the Heart*, North-Holland, Amsterdam, 1971.
10. Schuler G, Schwartz F, Hofmann M, Mehmel H, Manthey J, Maurer W, Rauch B, Herrmann HJ, Kubler W: Thrombolysis in acute myocardial infarction using intracoronary streptokinase. Assessment by thallium-201 scintigraphy. Circulation 66:658–664, 1982.
11. Schwarz F, Schuler G, Katus H, Hofmann M, Manthey J, Tillmanns H, Mehmel HC, Kubler W: Intracoronary thrombolysis in acute myocardial infarction: Duration of ischemia as a major determinant of late results after recanalization. Am J Cardiol 50:933–937, 1982.
12. Swan HJC, Shah PK, Rubin S: Role of vasodilators in the changing phases of acute myocardial infarction. Am Heart J 103:703, 1982.
13. Jennings RB, Reimer KA: Factors involved in salvaging ischemic myocardium: Effect of reperfusion of arterial blood. Circulation 68(I):I-25–I-36, 1983.

14. Kloner RA, Ellis SG, Lange R, Braunwald E: Studies of experimental coronary artery perfusion. Effects on infarct size, myocardial function, biochemistry, ultrastructure and microvascular damage. Circulation 68(I):I-8–I-15, 1983.

15. Schaper J, Schaper W: Reperfusion of ischemic myocardium: ultrastructural and histochemical aspects. J Am Coll Cardiol 1:1037–1046, 1983.

16. Ellis SG, Henschke CI, Sandor T, Wynne J, Braunwald E, Kloner RA: Time course of functional and biochemical recovery of myocardium salvaged by reperfusion. J Am Coll Cardiol 1:1047–1055, 1983.

17. Kloner RA, Ganote CE, Jennings RB: The "no reflow" phenomenon after temporary coronary occlusion in the dog. J Clin Invest 54:1496–1508, 1974.

18. Kloner RA, Rude RE, Carlson N, Maroko PR, DeBoer LWV, Braunwald E: Ultrastructural evidence of microvascular damage and myocardial cell injury after coronary artery occlusion: which comes first? Circulation 62:945–952, 1980.

19. Pirzada FA, Weiner JM, Hood WB: Experimental myocardial infarction. 14. Accelerated myocardial stiffening related to coronary reperfusion following ischemia. Chest 74:190–195, 1978.

20. Haendchen RV, Corday E, Torres M, Maurer G, Fishbein MC, Meerbaum S: Increased regional end-diastolic wall thickness early after reperfusion: A sign of irreversibly damaged myocardium. J Am Coll Cardiol 3:1444–1453, 1984.

21. Cerra FB, Lagos TZ, Montes M, Siegel JH: Hemorrhagic infarction: A reperfusion injury following prolonged myocardial ischemic anoxia. Surgery 78:95–104, 1975.

22. Fishbein MC, Y-Rit J, Lando U, Kanmatsuse K, Mercier JC, Ganz W: The relationship of vascular injury and myocardial hemorrhage to necrosis after reperfusion. Circulation 62:1274–1279, 1980.

23. McNamara JJ, Lacro RV, Yee M, Smith GT: Hemorrhagic infarction and coronary reperfusion. J Thorac Cardiovasc Surg 81:498–501, 1981.

24. Higginson LAJ, White F, Heggtveit HA, Sanders TM, Bloor CM, Covell JW: Determinants of myocardial hemorrhage after coronary reperfusion in the anesthetized dog. Circulation 65:62–69, 1982.

25. Agress CM, Jacobs HI, Maxwell JB, Clark WG, Kaplan L, Lederer M, Glasner HF: Intravenous trypsin in experimental myocardial infarction. Circ Research II(5):397, 1954.

26. The Multicenter Postinfarction Research Group: Risk stratification and survival after myocardial infarction. N Engl J Med 309(6):331, 1983.

27. Yusuf S, Collins R, Peto R, et al: Intravenous and intracoronary fibrinolytic therapy in acute myocardial infarction: overview of results on mortality, reinfarction, and side effects from 33 randomized trials. European Heart J 6:556, 1985.

28. Rentrop P, DeVivie ER, Karsch KR, Kreuzer H: Acute coronary occlusion with impending infarction as an angiographic complication relieved by guidewire canalization. Clin Cardiol 1:101, 1978.

29. Meyer J, Merx W, Schmitz HJ, et al: Percutaneous transluminal coronary an-

gioplasty immediately after intracoronary streptolysis of transmural myocardial infarction. Circulation 66:905, 1982.

30. Ganz W, Buchbinder N, Marcus H, et al: Intracoronary thrombolysis in evolving myocardial infarction. Am Heart J 101:4, 1981.

31. Mathey D, Kuck KH, Tilsner V, et al: Nonsurgical coronary artery recanalization in acute transmural myocardial infarction. Circulation 63:409, 1981.

32. Schroder R, Biamino G, vonLeitner ER, et al: Intravenous short-term infusion of streptokinase in acute myocardial infarction. Circulation 67:536, 1983.

33. Ganz W, Geft I, Shah PK, et al: Intravenous streptokinase in evolving myocardial infarction. Am J Cardiol 53:1209, 1984.

34. Simoons ML, Serruys PW, Brand M, et al: Improved survival after early thrombolysis in acute myocardial infarction. Lancet 2:578, 1985.

35. Kennedy JW, Ritchie JL, Davis KB, Fritz JK: Western Washington randomization trial of intracoronary streptokinase in acute myocardial infarction. N Engl J Med 309:1477, 1983.

36. Taylor GJ, Mikell FL, Moses W, et al: Intravenous versus intracoronary streptokinase therapy for acute myocardial infarction in community hospitals. Am J Cardiol 54:256, 1984.

37. Koran G, Weiss AT, Hasin Y, et al: Prevention of myocardial damage in acute myocardial ischemia by early treatment with intravenous streptokinase. N Engl J Med 313:1384, 1985.

38. Hillis LD, Borer J, Braunwald E, et al: High-dose intravenous streptokinase for acute myocardial infarction: preliminary results of a multicenter trial. J Am Coll Cardiol 6:957, 1985.

39. Monassier JP, Valeix B, Bory M, Guarino L, Labrunie P, Sainsous J, Coulbois PM, Ibrahim A: Intracoronary thrombolysis. "Paradoxical" increasing of chest and pain ST elevation during reperfusion (cooperative study). Eur Heart J 5(abstr): 25, 1984.

40. Sobel BE, Bergmann SR: Coronary thrombolysis: some unresolved issues. Am J Med 72:1, 1982.

41. Simoons ML, Brand M V/D, de Zwaan C, Verheugt FWA, Remme WJ, Serruys PW, Bar F, Res J, Krauss XH, Vermeer F: Improved survival after early thrombolysis in acute myocardial infarction. Lancet 2:578–582, 1985.

42. Effectiveness of intravenous thrombolytic therapy in acute myocardial infarction. Gruppo Italiano Per Lo Studio Della Streptochinasi Nell'infarto Miocardico (GISSI). Lancet 1:397, 1986.

43. Verstraete M, Bory M, Collen D: Randomized trial of intravenous recombinant tissue-type plasminogen activator vs. intravenous streptokinase in acute myocardial infarct. Report from the European Cooperative Study Group for Recombinant Tissue Type Plasminogen Activator. Lancet 2:842, 1985.

44. Marder VJ, Rothbard RL, Fitzpatrick PG, Francis CW: Rapid lysis of coronary artery thrombi with anisoylated plasminogen: streptokinase activator complex. Ann Intern Med 104:304, 1986.

5

Thrombolysis in Myocardial Infarction: The NHLBI Experience

Eugene R. Passamani
National Heart, Lung and Blood Institute
Bethesda, Maryland

I. INTRODUCTION

Coronary artery disease is a major U.S. public health problem that results each year in an estimated 540,000 deaths and 700,000 hospital admissions for acute myocardial infarction (1,2). Atherosclerosis involving the coronary arterial system begins in early adulthood and progresses over a rather lengthy asymptomatic period in middle age, ultimately resulting in symptoms beginning in the fourth and fifth decades. Coronary disease presents symptomatically with angina pectoris, sudden cardiac death, or acute myocardial infarction.

In recent years, the application of coronary arteriography in the early hours of myocardial infarction and the administration of thrombolytic agents have resulted in both a clearer understanding of the conversion from chronic stable coronary disease to acute myocardial infarction and an appreciation of the potential for thrombolytic therapy to favorably influence the course of myocardial infarction (3–6).

II. THROMBOLYSIS IN MYOCARDIAL INFARCTION

The National Heart, Lung, and Blood Institute (NHLBI), together with the Bureau of Biologics of the Food and Drug Administration, supported a 2-day workshop in November 1981 to review relevant data regarding the clinical application of thrombolytic therapy and to make recommendations regarding research initiatives that might clarify the indications for this innovative treatment (7). The workshop participants recommended the establishment of a clinical investigative group to design and carry out clinical trials that would clarify the role of thrombolytic therapy in patients with acute infarction. After favorable review by the NHLBI Cardiology Advisory Committee and Advisory Council, the institute established the Thrombolysis in Myocardial Infarction (TIMI) Study Group in July 1983. The group comprised 13 clinical sites and a variety of central support units (see Appendix). At that time, a number of investigators had already reported reperfusion results with intracoronary and intravenous streptokinase and, to a lesser extent, urokinase (6). In addition, a new generation of more fibrin-specific thrombolytic agents were being developed and would soon be available for clinical trials (8–10).

Design of a trial of thrombolytic therapy required careful resolution of a number of issues, including selection of a thrombolytic agent and the dose and route of administration. The TIMI investigators chose the intravenous route since this is the only method that might reach a majority of myocardial infarction victims in time to interrupt infarction. Choosing the thrombolytic agent was most difficult: Choice of streptokinase or urokinase could lead to results that might have been rendered moot by the development of a much more effective new thrombolytic agent, while choice of an untried new and theoretically better agent might lead to an enormous waste of effort should the new agent prove to be clinically ineffective or, worse, dangerous. The solution adopted was a series of investigations designed to clarify the relative efficacy of representatives of the conventional and new classes of thrombolytic agents followed by a more definitive investigation of the agent that appeared most promising (11–13).

From June 1984 to March 1986, six distinct investigations were carried out by the TIMI cooperative group, as displayed on Table 1. These investigations included comparative studies of streptokinase (SK) and recombinant tissue plasminogen activator (rt-PA), as well as a series of rt-PA dose response investigations culminating in Phase II, a trial designed to assess the combination of rt-PA and percutaneous transluminal coronary angioplasty

Table 1 TIMI Investigations, 1984–1986

Phase	Design				Results	
	Drug	Dose	Randomized	n	Reperfused at 90 min (%)	Average decrease fibrinogen (%)
Open-label 1984	rt-PA (G11021)	80 mg/3 hr (40,20,20)	No	47	68	29
Open-label 1984	SK	1.5 mU/1 hr	No	40	32	53
I	rt-PA (G11021)	80 mg/3 hr (40,20,20)	Yes	290	62	27
	SK	1.5 mU/1 hr			31	57
Open-label 1985						
A	rt-PA (G11035)	80 mg/3 hr (40,20,20)	No	48	45 (13)[a]	3
B	rt-PA (G11035)	100 mg/3 hr (60,20,20)	No	87	71 (24)[a]	8
C	rt-PA (G11035)	150 mg/6 hr (90,20,10 × 4)	No	65	76 (42)[a]	24

[a]30-min reperfusion.

(PTCA) in patients with acute myocardial infarction. The remainder of this chapter includes a discussion of the design and published findings from this series of investigations.

Design

The TIMI Phase I protocol involved coronary arteriography in patients in the very early hours of acute infarction followed by a double-blind randomized study of two thrombolytic drugs. Given the complexity of this protocol and the fact that only 45 patients with infarction had received rt-PA at the time TIMI investigations were about to begin (10), two open-label investigations were undertaken as a rehearsal for the randomized study. The first study, open-label rt-PA, involved 47 patients treated with known rt-PA; the second, open-label SK, involved 40 patients treated with known SK.

The designs of the open-label rt-PA and SK studies and TIMI Phase I, which followed these studies, were identical, with the exception that during Phase I patients were randomly assigned to receive rt-PA or SK and the assignment was masked. For each of these three separate investigations, patients entering cooperating hospitals with ischemic chest pain of at least 30-min duration and ST-segment elevation of at least 0.1 mV in at least two ECG leads, who were less than 76 years of age, without a history of coronary artery bypass surgery, and who appeared within 7 hr of the onset of chest pain were asked to participate in the trial. After informed consent had been obtained, patients were taken directly to the cardiac catheterization laboratory, arterial and venous access established, 5000 U of heparin given intravenously, left ventriculography performed in the right anterior oblique position, and coronary arteriography obtained with the infarct related artery studied last.

Thrombolytic therapy was initiated in those with more than 50% coronary stenosis after intracoronary administration of 200 μg of nitroglycerin. Genentech, Inc., supplied rt-PA (G11021), which was given over 3 hr, 40 mg in the first hour and 20 mg in each of the 2 subsequent hours. Hoescht-Roussel Pharmaceuticals and Kabi-Vitrum, A.B., supplied streptokinase; each SK patient was treated with 1.5 million U given over 1 hr. Coronary arteriography was repeated 10, 20, 30, 45, 60, 75, and 90 min after the initiation of thrombolytic therapy. Reperfusion was graded by investigators at the clinical units and subsequently by the radiographic core laboratory according to rigorously defined criteria, displayed in Table 2. The measurement of primary interest was the 90-min opacification of the infarct-related artery, 30 min after 1.5 million U of SK had been infused or after 50 mg of rt-PA had been given. The coagulation core laboratory provided measurements of fibrinogen and

Table 2   Definitions of Perfusion in the TIMI Trial

Grade 0 (no perfusion)
There is no antegrade flow beyond the point of occlusion.

Grade 1 (penetration without perfusion)
The contrast material passes beyond the area of obstruction but "hangs up" and fails to opacify the entire coronary bed distal to the obstruction for the duration of the cineangiographic filming sequence.

Grade 2 (partial perfusion)
The contrast material passes across the obstruction and opacifies the coronary bed distal to the obstruction. However, the rate of entry of contrast material into the vessel distal to the obstruction or its rate of clearance from the distal bed (or both) are perceptibly slower than its entry into or clearance from comparable areas not perfused by the previously occluded vessel—e.g., the opposite coronary artery or the coronary bed proximal to the obstruction.

Grade 3 (complete perfusion)
Antegrade flow into the bed distal to the obstruction occurs as promptly as antegrade flow into the bed proximal to the obstruction, and clearance of contrast material from the involved bed is as rapid as clearance from an uninvolved bed in the same vessel or the opposite artery.

other coagulation factors at baseline and after infusion of thrombolytic agents. Patients were, thereafter, managed according to general TIMI guidelines, including heparin anticoagulation until recatheterization at hospital discharge whereupon each patient was placed on aspirin and dipyridamole.

III.   OPEN-LABEL rt-PA: RESULTS

A total of 47 patients entered the TIMI open-label rt-PA study (12). Thirty-seven (79%) were found to have total occlusion (grade 0,1) of the infarct-related artery at baseline. The average time from onset of symptoms to initiation of rt-PA infusion was 289 min, the delay due in large part to cardiac catheterization. Of these 37 patients, 25 (68%) demonstrated coronary reperfusion at 90 min after 50 mg of the total dose of 80 mg had been infused. A total of 21 of the 25 reperfused patients underwent arteriography at hospital discharge at which time 14 (67%) had persistently patent infarct-related arteries and 7 (33%) did not. In the 12 patients noted to have a persistently closed infarct-related artery at 90 min, six did not have a hospital discharge study; in the six studied, four had patent infarct-related arteries. Nine of 10 patients found to have open infarct-related arteries at baseline were studied before discharge and eight (89%) were found to have persistently open coronary arteries.

During the hospitalization, six patients (13%) died and 7 (15%) were judged to have evidence of reinfarction. Modest declines in fibrinogen (29% ± 16) were noted. Seven of 47 (15%) were noted to have evidence of a major (>5 g/dl) decrease in hemoglobin. Hematoma formation and bleeding at the catheterization sites were responsible for most of these episodes. Ten patients (21%) were given blood transfusions. Thus, this initial TIMI investigation demonstrated that intravenous infusion of 80 mg of rt-PA (G11021) given over 3 hr resulted in reperfusion in approximately two-thirds of patients found to have closed infarct-related arteries at baseline. Modest changes in plasma levels of fibrinogen were observed. Bleeding at the catheterization site was common, and 10 patients ultimately required blood transfusions.

IV.   OPEN-LABEL STREPTOKINASE: RESULTS

A total of 40 patients entered the TIMI open-label SK study, an average of 270 min after onset of chest pain (11). At 90 min, 11 of 34 patients (32%) noted to have baseline occlusion (grade 0,1) were successfully reperfused, ½ hr after 1.5 million U of SK had been infused. Six of 11 successfully reperfused patients underwent arteriography at hospital discharge at which time five (83%) had persistently patent infarct-related arteries. Hospital discharge catheterization was carried out in 13 of 23 patients who were not reperfused at 90 min; 7 (54%) were open at discharge.

Three of these 40 patients died during the hospitalization (8%). Six patients (15%) required transfusion during hospitalization; bleeding at the catheterization site and hematoma formations were responsible for most bleeding complications. Substantial reductions were noted in fibrinogen (53%) after the administration of streptokinase. In summary, this initial TIMI streptokinase investigation demonstrated reperfusion in approximately one-third of patients with closed infarct-related arteries at entry. Substantial reductions were noted in the concentration of fibrinogen. This low rate of induced reperfusion became part of a very wide variation in reported reperfusion rates with streptokinase and was, in fact, a harbinger of Phase I findings.

V.   TIMI PHASE I

During TIMI Phase I, which lasted from August 1984 to February 1985, 290 patients were randomized in a double-blind fashion to intravenous streptokinase, 1.5 million U given over 1 hr, or rt-PA 80 mg given over 3 hr (40 mg the first hour and 20 mg in each of 2 subsequent hours) (13). The treatment assignment was masked by giving each patient two infusions (either SK and rt-PA placebo or SK placebo and rt-PA). A total of 113 patients assigned rt-PA and 119 patients assigned SK had completely closed (grade 0,1) infarct-related arteries at baseline. The TIMI central radiographic laboratory, which was not aware of clinical details or local interpretation, noted that 62% of rt-PA patients and 31% of SK patients had an open infarct-related artery at 90 min (16). This difference is exceedingly unlikely to have arisen by chance (p < 0.001) and was the reason TIMI I was stopped before the scheduled termination date (13). The percentages reported in the preliminary communication were based on local clinical readings and thus differ minimally from the central readings noted above (13).

Death during the hospital course occurred in seven (5%) of patients in the rt-PA group and 12 (8%) in patients assigned to the SK group. Clinical reinfarction occurred in 13 and 10%, respectively, of the rt-PA and the SK groups. Substantial differences were noted in coagulation factors with, for example, reduction in fibrinogen levels by 27 and 57%, respectively, for rt-PA and SK after the thrombolytic infusion. During hospitalization, transfusions were administered to 41 (29%) of patients in the rt-PA group and 40 (27%) of patients in the streptokinase group. Bleeding or hematoma formation was noted at the catheterization site in more than 80% of rt-PA and SK patients.

Thus, TIMI Phase I, in a double-blind randomized comparison of intravenous streptokinase versus intravenous rt-PA demonstrated that rt-PA is approximately twice as effective as SK in opening closed coronary arteries and results in less fibrinogen degradation. The combination of hemorrhage at the catheterization site and phlebotomy resulted in transfusion of nearly one-third of these patients. A small nonsignificant difference in mortality was observed.

VI. OPEN LABEL: 1985

A new preparation of predominantly single-chain rt-PA (G11035) became available in 1985. The TIMI investigators, in preparation for a long-term trial using rt-PA, conducted a series of investigations, summarized in Table 1. These studies were designed to determine the optimum dose and rate of administration by using a protocol similar to that used in Phase I. Patients satisfying similar entrance and exclusion criteria were taken to the cardiac catheterization laboratory for visualization of coronary anatomy. In those with an occluded infarct-related artery, three series of patients were treated with three increasing doses of new rt-PA (14,15). A total of 48 patients were treated with 80 mg (40 mg during the first hour and 20 mg in each of 2 subsequent hours). Eighty-seven patients were treated with 100 mg (60 mg with a 6-mg bolus in the first hour and 20 mg in each of 2 subsequent hours) and 65 patients were treated with 150 mg (90 mg with a 9-mg bolus over the first hour, 20 mg over the second hour, and 10 mg in each of 4 subsequent hours). A substantial increase in 30-min arterial patency led to the choice of 150 mg as the dose to be used in TIMI Phase II. In addition, during this series of investigations, catheterization was repeated at 18 to 48 hr to determine whether angioplasty could be performed. In aggregate, approximately two-thirds of the patients given rt-PA within 7 hr of onset of chest pain have coronary anatomy that is technically feasible for PTCA at 18 to 48 hr. Approximately one-sixth have insufficient coronary narrowing to require PTCA, and the remaining one-sixth are technically impossible (16).

VII. TIMI PHASE II

As a consequence of TIMI results and findings from other investigations of thrombolytic therapy in patients with acute infarction (17–19), the final Phase II TIMI protocol will involve the design displayed in Figure 1. All patients presenting to cooperating hospitals within 4 hr of onset of chest pain with elevated ST segments in the absence of the exclusion criteria will be given 150 mg of rt-PA over 6 hr. Patients will be randomized to no PTCA unless clinically required or PTCA if at all possible. Nested in the overall trial are two subtrials: 1) TIMI IIa to be carried out at seven sites in which all patients are given rt-PA and randomized to one of three groups, PTCA carried out immediately, PTCA carried out at 18–48 hr and, finally, no PTCA unless clinically indicated, and 2) TIMI IIb to be carried out at 17 sites, which includes a factorial design. Patients believed clinically unable to tolerate intravenous beta blockers will be randomized to PTCA at 18 to 48 hr or PTCA only if clinically required. Patients able to tolerate intravenous beta blockade will be assigned among four treatment groups: PTCA at 18 to 48 hr versus no PTCA and acute intravenous beta blockade versus deferred beta blockade. The primary endpoint for the overall comparison of PTCA versus no PTCA in rt-PA-treated patients will be survival to 6 weeks free of recurrent infarction. A number of secondary endpoints will be examined, including mortality at hospital discharge, 6 weeks and 1 year; resting and exercise left ventricular function; hemorrhagic events; and changes in coagulation factors.

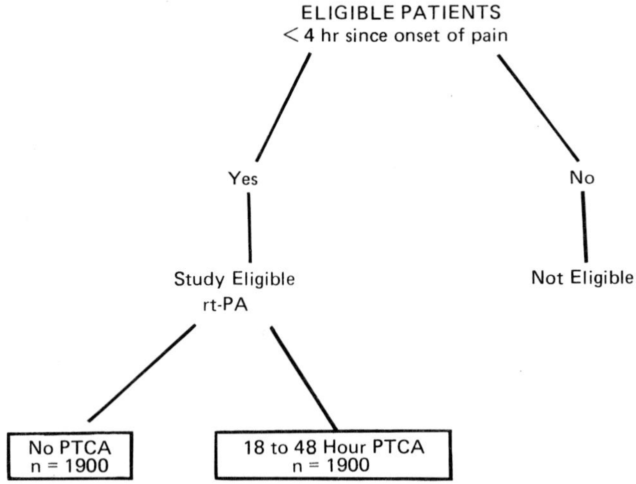

Figure 1   TIMI Phase II design. Expected recruitment = 3800 patients.

VIII. CONCLUSION

A revolution is occurring in the treatment of patients with acute myocardial infarction. This has been driven in part by the development of a new generation of fibrin-specific thrombolytic drugs, which are quite effective given intravenously and offer the potential of early reperfusion leading to interruption of myocardial infarction. A number of important research questions remain, including: the proper mix of adjunctive pharmacological therapy such as beta blockers, calcium channel antagonists, and possibly free radical scavengers; whether medical therapy such as antiplatelet or anticoagulants drugs is sufficient to prevent recurrence of coronary thrombosis; and the time interval beyond which reperfusion is ineffective and the means whereby patients at high risk of recurrence can be selected for more definitive and invasive therapy such as percutaneous transluminal coronary angioplasty and coronary artery bypass graft surgery.

Early self-referral and expeditious delivery of thrombolytic and other adjunctive therapies are essential if this major advance in the understanding of myocardial infarction is to be translated into reduced morbidity and mortality in patients with coronary disease.

APPENDIX

Thrombolysis in Myocardial Infarction

Clinical Sites

Brown University: David Williams, M.D.
University of Massachusetts: Joel Gore, M.D.
Mayo Clinic: James Chesebro, M.D.
Baylor College of Medicine: Robert Roberts, M.D.
Albert Einstein: Hiltrud Mueller, M.D.
George Washington University: Alan Ross, M.D.
Columbia University: Eric Powers, M.D.
Cornell Medical Center: Jeffrey Borer, M.D.
Yale University: Charles Francis, M.D.
Harvard University: John Markis, M.D.
University of Texas: James Willerson, M.D.
Washington University: Philip Ludbrook, M.D.
Boston University: Thomas Ryan, M.D.

Central Units

Data Coordinating Center: Maryland Medical Research Institute, Genell
   Knatterud, Ph.D.

Drug Distribution Center: Albuquerque, VA Hospital, Michael Kovach

Central Laboratories

Radiographic: University of Washington, Harold Dodge, M.D.
Radionuclear: Yale University, Barry Zaret, M.D.
Coagulation: Temple University, A. Koneti Rao, M.D.
Electrocardiographic: George Washington University, Alan Ross, M.D.
Pathology: National Heart, Lung and Blood Institute, NIH, William
   Roberts, M.D.

Steering Committee Chairman: Harvard University, Eugene Braunwald,
   M.D.

NHLBI Program Office: Eugene Passamani, M.D., Thomas Robertson,
   M.D, and Patrice Nickens, M.D.

REFERENCES

1. National Center for Health Statistics: *Monthly Vital Statistics Report,* vol. 33, no. 13, September 26, 1985.
2. National Center for Health Statistics: *Detailed Diagnosis and Procedures for Patients Discharged from Short-Stay Hospitals, United States, 1984, Data from The National Health Survey Series,* vol. 13, no. 86.
3. Laffel GL, Braunwald E: Thrombolytic therapy: A new strategy for treatment of acute myocardial infarction. N Engl J Med 311:710–716, 770–775, 1984.
4. DeWood MA, Spores J, Notske R, et al: Prevalence of total coronary occlusion during the early hours of transmural myocardial infarction. N Engl J Med 303:897–902, 1980.
5. Rentrop P, Blanke H, Karsh KR, et al: Selective intracoronary thrombolysis in acute myocardial infarction and unstable angina pectoris. Circulation 63:307–317, 1981.
6. Rentrop PK: Thrombolytic therapy in patients with acute myocardial infarction. Circulation 71:627–631, 1985.
7. Passamani, ER (guest editor): Limitation of infarct size with thrombolytic agents. Proceedings of the workshop, November 9–10, 1981. National Institutes of Health, Bethesda, Maryland. American Heart Association Monograph no. 97, 1983.
8. Collen D, Verstraete M: Systemic thrombolytic therapy of acute myocardial infarction? Circulation 68:462–465, 1983.
9. Van de Werf F, Ludbrook PA, Bergmann SR, et al: Coronary thrombolysis with tissue-type plasminogen activator in patients with evolving myocardial infarction. N Engl J Med 310:609–613, 1984.
10. Collen D, Topol EJ, Tiefenbrunn AS, et al: Coronary thrombolysis with recombinant human tissue-type plasminogen activator: A prospective, randomized, placebo-controlled trial. Circulation 70:1012–1017, 1984.
11. Hillis LD, Borer J, Braunwald E, et al: High-dose intravenous streptokinase for acute myocardial infarction: Preliminary results of a multicenter trial. J Am Coll Cardiol 6(5):957–962, 1985.
12. Williams DO, Borer J, Braunwald E, et al: Intravenous recombinant tissue-type plasminogen activator in patients with acute myocardial infarction: A report from the NHLBI thrombolysis in myocardial infarction trial. Circulation 73(2):338–346, 1986.
13. The TIMI Study Group: The Thrombolysis in Myocardial Infarction (TIMI) Trial. Phase I findings. N Engl J Med 312:932–936, 1985.
14. Mueller H: Different fibrinolytic potencies of two forms of recombinant tissue-type plasminogen activator. NHLBI Thrombolysis in Myocardial Infarction Trial. Clin Res 34:631A, 1986.
15. Rao AK: Differential effects in vivo of predominantly single chain and double chain recombinant tissue plasminogen activator on plasma fibrinogen and fibrinolytic system. Clin Res 34:337A, 1986.

16. Braunwald E: *TIMI Update*. Presented at the Scientific Sessions of the American College of Cardiology March 10, 1986.
17. Verstraete M, Bory M, Collen D, et al: Randomized trial of intravenous recombinant tissue-type plasminogen activator versus intravenous streptokinase in acute myocardial infarction. Lancet 578–581, 1985.
18. GISSI: Effectiveness of intravenous thrombolytic treatment in acute myocardial infarction. Lancet 377–401, 1986.
19. The I.S.A.M. Study Group: A prospective trial of intravenous streptokinase in acute myocardial infarction (I.S.A.M.). N Engl J Med 314:1465–1471, 1986.

6

Myocardial Infarction: Thrombolysis and Angioplasty

Eric J. Topol and William W. O'Neill
University of Michigan Medical School
Ann Arbor, Michigan

In the vast majority of patients with evolving myocardial infarction, the culprit coronary artery contains both intraluminal thrombus and a significant atherosclerotic intimal plaque (1,2). Methods to achieve effective, complete, and sustained myocardial perfusion, therefore, must address both the underlying thrombotic and atherosclerotic processes. In this chapter, we will discussion reperfusion therapy using the combination of intravenous fibrinolysis and balloon percutaneous transluminal coronary angioplasty (PTCA).

I. PATHOPHYSIOLOGY

Although Herrick described the phenomenon in 1912 (3), coronary angiographic, pathological, and intraoperative studies in the past 5 years (4–7) have led to the acceptance that thrombotic occlusion is the immediate event responsible for curtailment of coronary blood flow. The pathogenesis of the thrombus appears to be related to plaque disruption, characterized by a tear in the fibrous cap of the plaque (8,9). As a result of this de novo intimal dissection, platelets are activated and thromboplastin is released. Thrombin formed in such a way leads to further amplification of platelet activation and development of fibrin. All of this takes place at the site of an atherosclerotic plaque, which at autopsy has been found to be high grade (>75% reduction of cross-sectional area) in approximately 85% of patients with acute myocardial infarction (10). In addition to understanding the pathophysiology of coronary thrombosis, experimental studies have demonstrated the clearcut time dependency of myocardial reperfusion in achieving salvage of jeopardized myocardium (11).

II. INTRACORONARY AND INTRAVENOUS STREPTOKINASE

The optimal approach to recanalization of the occluded coronary artery is currently under intense scrutiny and has rapidly evolved over the past few years. In the early 1980s intracoronary streptokinase became popular as a technique to restore flow to the occluded coronary artery and it has been shown to be 75% effective in achieving this goal (12). The time delay with this therapy is significant, usually 1.5 to 2 hr. This may explain why randomized, controlled studies showed little or no evidence of preserved ventricular function with intracoronary streptokinase (12–14).

With the intravenous route of administering thrombolytic agents, there exists potential for more rapid initiation of therapy and wide-scale application. The largest randomized, controlled study using intravenous thrombolysis was performed in Italy (15). In this GISSI trial of nearly 12,000 patients, there was an overall 19% reduction in mortality for patients treated with streptokinase, compared to those randomized to conventional therapy. However, in the streptokinase patients there was a 100% increase in the incidence of reinfarction compared to conventionally treated patients during the first 21 days after hospital admission. Similar results of increased reinfarction among patients receiving thrombolytic therapy compared to controls were obtained in the Netherlands Inter-University Trial (16).

Pooled angiographic studies with intravenous streptokinase at the doses employed in these trials (1.5 million U over 30–60 min) have shown a 50% infarct vessel patency rate (12,17). Since the clinical introduction of recombinant tissue-type plasminogen activator (rt-PA) in 1984, combined studies suggest its patency rate to be 70% or greater (18–22). With the increased efficacy of rt-PA for achieving recanalization, there is even higher potential for reinfarction. This concern for reinfarction and rethrombosis accounted for the secondary goal of definitive recanalization. In order to assure sustained infarct vessel patency, treatment of the underlying plaque with PTCA or surgical revascularization became a logical next step (23).

III. CORONARY ANGIOPLASTY

In parallel with the development of intravenous clot-selective fibrinolysis with rt-PA, experience with coronary angioplasty was rapidly advancing. Since its introduction in 1977, percutaneous balloon dilation of a high-grade coronary atherosclerotic stenosis has gained increased acceptance in the management of angina and, in particular, underlying single-vessel coronary artery disease. It was first applied in acute myocardial infarction in the early 1980s at a time when only nonsteerable balloon catheters were available. Meyer and co-workers studied the role of PTCA after intracoronary streptokinase and found that successful dilation could be achieved in 17 of 21 patients who had responded to fibrinolytic therapy (24). Many other investigators confirmed the safety and feasibilty of PTCA after intracoronary and intravenous strep-tokinase (25–28).

Hartzler et al. expanded the use of PTCA in myocardial infarction by applying this procedure to patients with an occluded infarct vessel who had not received thrombolytic treatment. This primary rather than adjunctive role of PTCA has led to successful recanalization in over 90% of 400 patients treated by Hartzler and co-workers (personal communication). With mechanical recanalization therapy that was safe and effective, a new alternative strategy was available for patients who failed fibrinolytic therapy or for those in whom such therapy was contraindicated. Further, in places where an experienced PTCA team is readily available and the patient can be treated quickly, in many patients direct mechanical therapy may be performed in less time than it would take for intravenous fibrinolytic therapy to lyse the coronary thrombus. This approach would avoid the potential bleeding risks associated with lytic therapy.

IV. PTCA: TECHNICAL CONSIDERATIONS

Clinical experience has allowed adaption of the PTCA technique for patients with total or subtotal occlusion of the infarct-related artery. Time is crucial, so patients are treated as soon as possible after symptom onset. Baseline coronary arteriography is performed to identify the infarct-related artery, assess the extent of angiographic collaterals, and exclude patients with lesions not suitable for PTCA. Patients with subtotal occlusion have PTCA performed in standard fashion with steerable guidewires. Patients with total coronary occlusion have clot perforation performed with guidewires of varying stiffness and dimensions (0.014 to 0.018 in.). Often guidewire penetration of the thrombus alone results in partial reperfusion, manifest by reperfusion arrhythmias and chest pain relief. Although intraluminal thrombosis is present in most infarct-related arteries subject to PTCA, there is usually only angiographic evidence of a small or no filling defect after the procedure, which can generally decrease the translesional gradient to less than 20 mm Hg and the luminal stenosis to less than 50%. Occasionally, one may see distal pruning of a vessel that supports embolization or an artery that is filled with multiple negative defects, suggestive of extensive and persistent thrombotic material.

With intravenous thrombolytic agents administered prior to study, the majority of patients have subtotal coronary occlusion at initial angiography. These cases are now more similar to elective procedures with potential for abrupt closure, necessitating surgical backup. If coronary dissection occurs, as manifest by recurrent chest pain, high translesional gradients, and visible intimal tears, patients are referred for immediate bypass surgery.

Criteria for selection of patients for PTCA in acute myocardial infarction are important and leave room for subjectivity and individual operator judgment. In our experience, suitable candidates for PTCA include patients with: 1) a clearly demonstrable infarct-related artery, 2) absence of severe, diffuse disease of the involved vessel with multiple stenoses and intimal irregularities, 3) a lesion that appears to be accessible to current dilation hardware, and 4) absence of left main anatomy (stenosis >60%) or >90% proximal lesions of both the left anterior descending and circumflex arteries. If a coronary artery has partially or fully recanalized after thrombolysis, a ''roadmap'' is set up that facilitates the introduction of the guidewire and dilation catheter. Only the infarct-related artery is approached with PTCA during the acute procedure. Previous studies have demonstrated the hazard associated with dilating the critical lesions in the noninfarct vessel(s) acutely (Hartzler, personal communication).

V. CORONARY ANGIOPLASTY VERSUS
INTRACORONARY STREPTOKINASE

To evaluate the efficacy of thrombolytic therapy with intracoronary streptokinase compared to direct PTCA, we performed a randomized, prospective clinical trial (29). The intent of this study was to determine whether immediate diminution of the underlying residual stenosis was more effective than thrombolytic therapy alone in preserving ventricular function and lessening postprocedure ischemic complications. We found that 56 of 72 patients (77%) presenting within 6 hr of symptom onset were technically suitable for PTCA. The number of eligible patients was higher than in earlier studies, such as that of Meyer et al. (24), and this reflects improvements in catheter technology and a willingness to attempt to recanalize completely occluded arteries. Of the 56 patients technically suitable for PTCA, 29 were randomized to PTCA and 27 to intracoronary streptokinase. The time from onset of symptoms to treatment and time to reperfusion were comparable for the two groups. Reperfusion of the occluded artery occurred in 85% of both treatment groups. Residual stenosis was significantly lowered for patients treated with PTCA (Figure 1). The most important finding was that patients treated with PTCA had significantly better preservation of global (Figure 2) and regional (Figure 3) myocardial function.

We concluded that the underlying residual stenosis after thrombolytic therapy prevented maximal improvement of ventricular function. It remained unclear whether this was related to a reduction of infarct size or augmentation of coronary blood flow. The role of PTCA in limiting infarct size was studied (30) in 40 patients in this trial (18 streptokinase, 22 PTCA) by comparing enzymatic infarct size, which showed no difference despite a mean ejection fraction increase of $8 \pm 11\%$ for PTCA patients and only $0.7 \pm 4\%$ for streptokinase treated patients ($p < 0.02$). Although there are limitations of

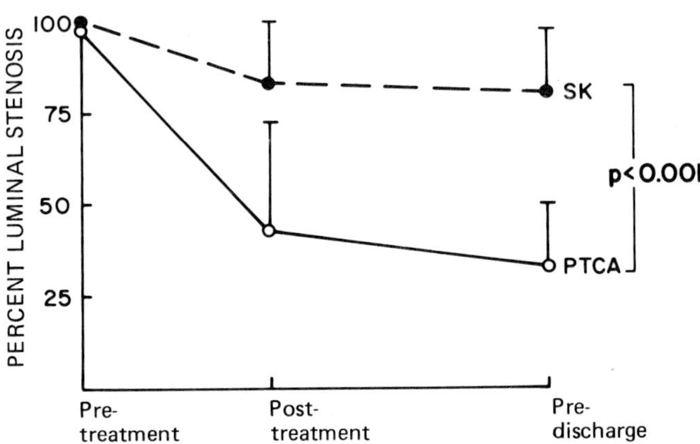

Figure 1	Difference in infarct vessel lesion stenosis in patients randomized to percutaneous transluminal coronary angioplasty (PTCA) or intracoronary streptokinase (SK) before and after acute therapy and at repeat study 7 to 10 days. (From Ref. 29.)

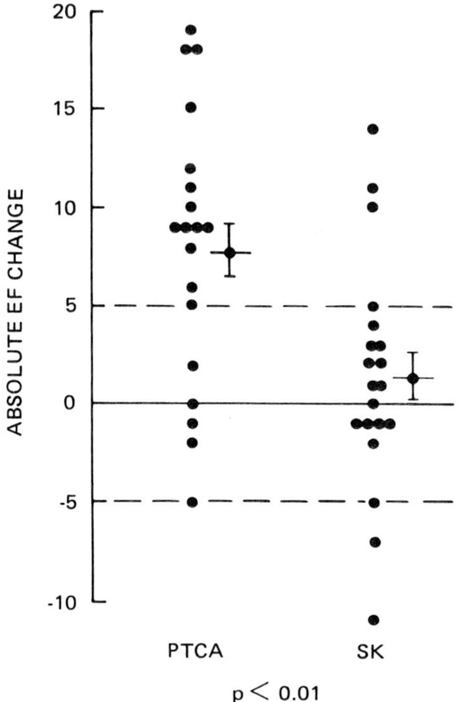

Figure 2   Global left ventricular ejection fraction of patients randomized to PTCA or intracoronary streptokinase. Values are the differences in ejection fraction for each patient with acute and followup ventriculograms. (From Ref. 29.)

enzymatic infarct size in the setting of reperfusion, the absence of any gross differences suggested that this was not the mechanism for improved ventricular function.

During this trial, we analyzed coronary sinus flow changes in 13 patients with anterior MI, presenting with complete left anterior descending (LAD) artery occlusion (31). Only patients with an LAD stenosis $\leq 50\%$ had significantly increased greater cardiac vein flow after reperfusion (Figure 4). This finding suggests that patients treated with thrombolytic therapy alone may not have effective restoration of coronary blood flow. This is consistent with the observation of Brown et al. that intracoronary streptokinase only partially lyses the obstructing thrombus, resulting in inadequate recanalization in 50% of cases (32).

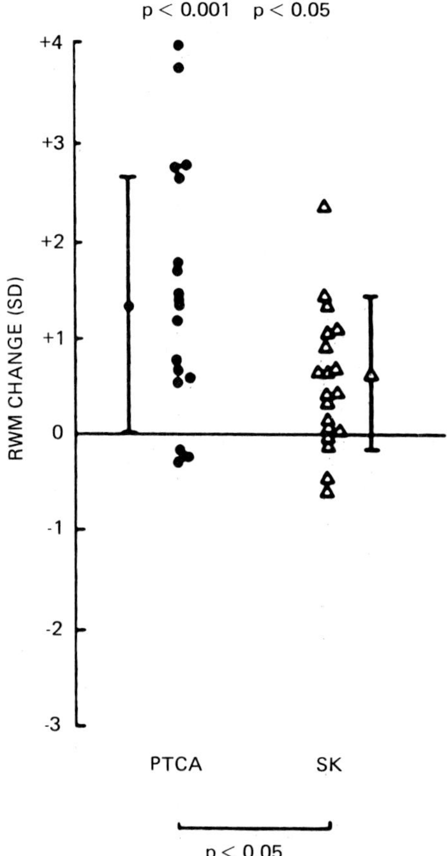

Figure 3   Changes in regional infarct-zone wall motion as determined using the centerline chord method for patients randomized to intracoronary streptokinase or PTCA. Values plotted represent the difference in regional wall motion, expressed as standard deviation units, from acute to followup ventriculography. (From Ref. 29.)

We further analyzed the impact of residual stenosis on exercise-induced periinfarction ischemia in 28 patients who underwent exercise tomographic scintigraphy during this trial (33). Patients treated with PTCA had a significantly lower incidence of exercise-induced periinfarct zone ischemia (9% vs. 60%; $p < 0.05$). When luminal stenosis after therapy was correlated to exercise-induced ischemia, only patients with residual stenosis $\geq 50\%$ had

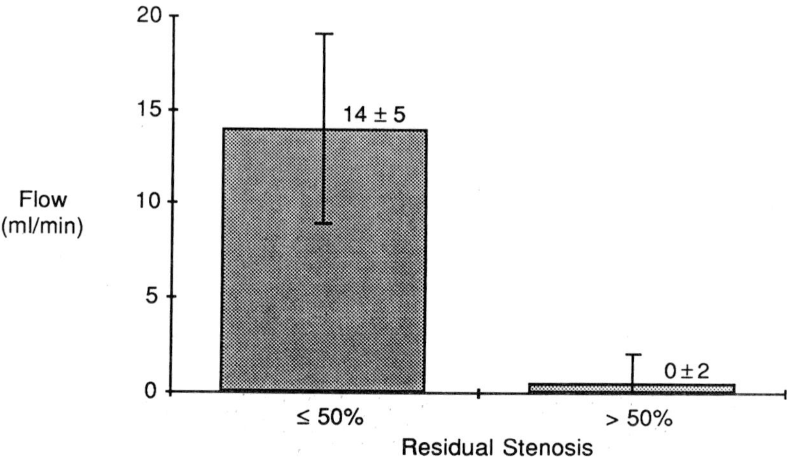

Figure 4   Change in coronary sinus flow, as determined by great cardiac vein (GCV) thermodilution in 13 patients with left anterior descending artery infarction. Only patients with a residual stenosis of <50% had an increment of GCV flow.

provocable ischemia (Figure 5). These three small substudies provided additional understanding about the importance and mechanism of a high-grade residual stenosis after thrombolytic therapy. From our pilot data, it appeared that it was important to achieve <50% residual stenosis in order to improve coronary blood flow, prevent exercise-induced ischemia, and augment ventricular function. Whether or not it is essential to achieve more complete recanalization immediately remains an unanswered question.

VI.   INTRAVENOUS STREPTOKINASE AND CORONARY ANGIOPLASTY

The study outlined above relied on baseline coronary angiography before therapy could be applied. A blind, empirical approach using intravenous thrombolytic therapy is the most rapid and practical means of achieving recanalization. Except in select circumstances where coronary angiography and angioplasty can be performed more quickly than it would take for an intravenous lytic agent to work, or in patients who have significant risks for bleeding, the first line of therapy should probably include intravenous thrombolysis. In the event that pharmacological thrombolysis proves suboptimal, the timing and nature of definitive therapy becomes a critical issue.

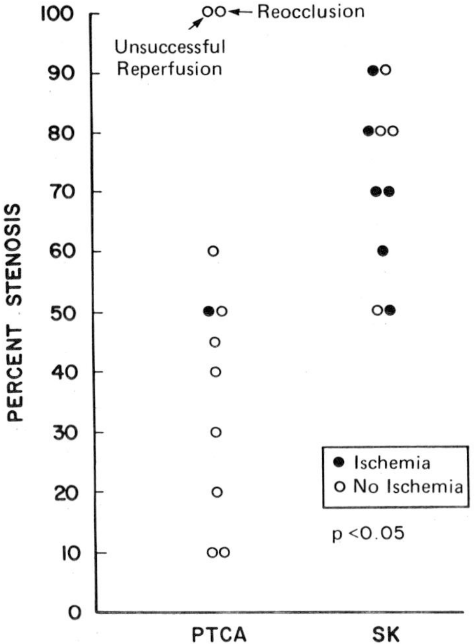

Figure 5   The impact of therapy and residual stenosis after acute myocardial infarction on exercise-induced periinfarct-zone ischemia. The residual stenosis of 28 randomized PTCA or intracoronary streptokinase-treated patients are shown. Closed circles represent ischemia confirmed by tomographic thallium scintigraphy. Half of patients with SK versus 6% of patients with PTCA therapy exhibited periinfarct ischemia. (From Ref. 33.)

For these reasons we studied the combination of intravenous streptokinase with emergent coronary angioplasty, known as "streptoplasty" in some institutions. In our first experience of 34 consecutive patients, therapy was initiated at 2.6 ± 1.3 hr after onset of symptoms (34). Therapy was begun at outlying, rural community hospitals, and helicopter transport was used to get patients to our cardiac catheterization facility very rapidly. Angiography, performed at 70 ± 14 min after therapy, documented persistent occlusion of the infarct vessel in 38% of patients, a high-grade residual stenosis in 52% of patients, and less than a 50% residual stenosis in 10% of patients. Of the 34 patients studied, 29 underwent immediate PTCA. There were only two patients with a ≥50% residual lesion who did not receive PTCA therapy. One of these had an unidentifiable infarct vessel (critical lesions in both the right and circumflex coronary arteries), and the other had a distal circumflex artery stenosis that was deemed not suitable for PTCA. Angioplasty was successful in 28 of 29 (96%) of patients, including 12 of 13 patients with persistent occlusion and all 16 patients who had recanalized after streptokinase therapy. Blinded review of paired left ventriculograms, obtained during the acute procedure and at 7–10-day followup, showed significant improvement in global left ventricular ejection fraction from 53 ± 12 to 59 ± 13% (p < 0.002). Of note, there was substantial recovery of regional and global function in those patients who had failed therapy with intravenous streptokinase. Thus, this observation demonstrated the potential for PTCA therapy to promote functional recovery even in patients who failed thrombolysis. This particular finding also reinforced the potential need for emergency cardiac catheterization, because this procedure would not only provide infarct vessel patency data, but also permit immediate mechanical recanalization of patients with persistent occlusion.

To determine the efficiency of PTCA with or without thrombolysis, we compared our experience with direct PTCA to our experience with sequential streptokinase and PTCA (35). A comparison of the key features of each approach is presented in Table 1. In 90 patients (47 direct, 43 sequential), there was a more significant improvement of global and regional function for patients treated sequentially (Figure 6). The PTCA success rate was similar in the two groups, 93% for direct and 96% for streptoplasty. All of the patients received heparin (intravenously for 1 week), aspirin, and dipyridamole. Even

Table 1   Bleeding Complications

	Sequential (n = 43)	Direct (n = 47)
Significant (>250 cc)	10	12
Site		
Periaccess	18	15
UGI	3	2
GU	1	0
Hemoptysis	1	0
Transfused (≥2 μ PRBC)	8	10

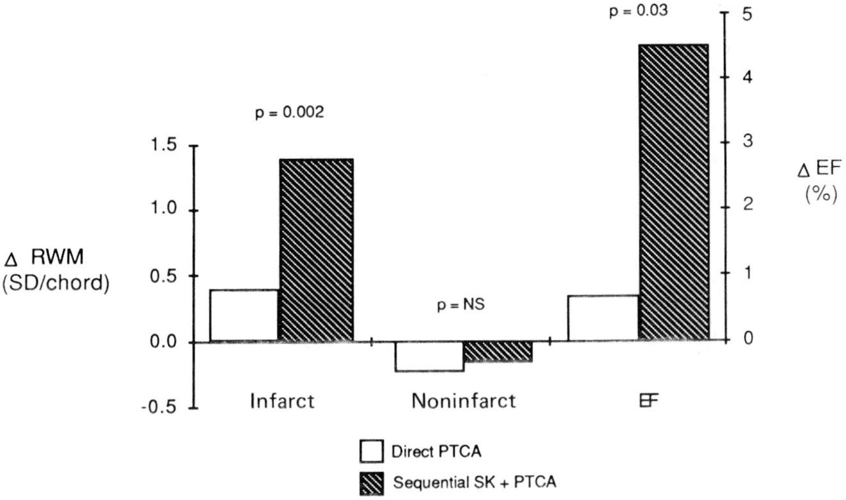

Figure 6 The difference in infarct-zone/noninfarct-zone regional wall motion and global ejection fraction in patients treated with sequential intravenous streptokinase and PTCA compared to PTCA only for acute myocardial infarction. There was a significant augmentation of infarct-zone wall motion, expressed as standard deviation units per chord; for sequentially treated patients, no difference in noninfarct-zone function. Global ejection fraction was significantly improved in the sequential compared to direct PTCA patients.

though half of the patients received intravenous streptokinase and developed a systemic lytic state, bleeding complications were similar in the two groups (Table 1). This supports the important etiological role of invasive punctures, heparin, and antiplatelet therapy for bleeding complications.

Our overall experience with intravenous streptokinase has pointed out major deficiencies of this therapy. Arterial reperfusion was achieved in only 59% (53 of 90) patients, and the presence of a marked fibrinolytic state mandated that femoral sheath access had to be maintained for at least 36 hr. There were substantial complications, including a 12% incidence of severe hypotension during drug infusion, bleeding complications requiring transfusion of at least two units of packed red cells in 18 patients, and a massive retroperitoneal hematoma in one patient. A more effective and clot-selective agent certainly held much promise for improved reperfusion results.

Table 2   Comparison of PTCA With and Without Thrombolysis

	Sequential SK + PTCA	Direct PTCA
Time	Rapid initiation	Obligatory delay
Rationale	Empiric	Tailored
Baseline angiogram	"Roadmap"	Cutoff
Fibrinogen breakdown	Severe	None

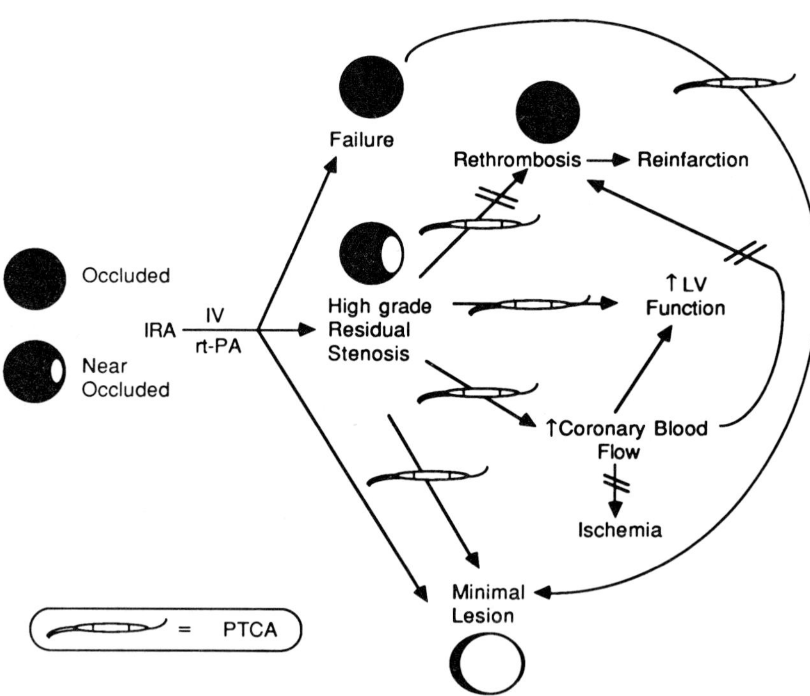

Figure 7   Potential mechanisms of coronary angioplasty benefit after t-PA therapy include decrease in the residual stenosis, successful recanalization of patients who fail thrombolysis, improvement of coronary blood flow, augmentation of myocardial infarction, and prevention of reocclusion.

VII. TISSUE PLASMINOGEN ACTIVATOR AND CORONARY ANGIOPLASTY

The potential mechanisms for PTCA benefit after intravenous t-PA are presented in Figure 7.

In the first multicenter trial of recombinant t-PA (18), a subset studied at one institution probed the effect of PTCA on all patients who had recanalized and were suitable candidates (36). Of 20 patients in this pilot trial, seven had successful t-PA and PTCA, or what we now term "plasminoplasty," six exhibited patency after t-PA but were not candidates or failed PTCA, and seven failed t-PA. In this small, nonrandomized trial, a significant improvement of infarct-zone wall motion was noted only in the successful plasminoplasty group by serial two-dimensional echocardiography (Figure 8). The results of this study coupled with those of the randomized intracoronary streptokinase and PTCA trial suggested a pivotal role of PTCA for preservation of myocardial function and served as the impetus for future trials.

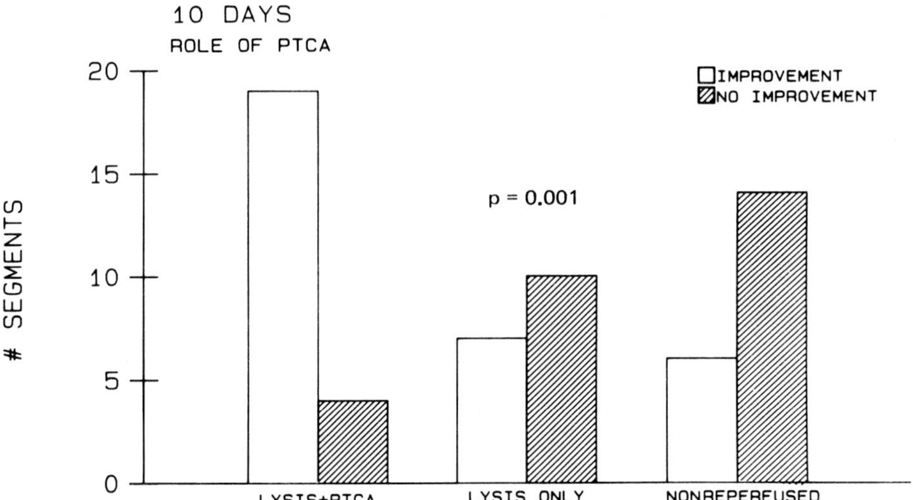

Figure 8   Change in regional wall motion, as determined by two-dimensional echocardiography, for patients who had t-PA and successful PTCA therapy, t-PA alone with perfusion, and failed t-PA therapy. Only patients with combined thrombolysis and PTCA treatment showed a significant improvement of infarct-zone wall motion. (From Ref. 36.)

A randomized, placebo-controlled trial of intravenous t-PA and PTCA was conducted at the University of Michigan in late 1985 (37) as part of another multicenter trial. Fifty patients were enrolled to receive t-PA (G11035) (1.25 mg/kg IV over 3 hr) or placebo using a 3:1 randomization scheme. At 120 min after therapy, infarct vessel patency was 84% in the t-PA group (32 of 38 patients) compared to 17% (two of 12 patients) in placebo-treated patients (p < 0.001). Of 32 patients with a patent vessel after t-PA, 28 were suitable for a second randomization to either immediate (15 patients) or no (13 patients) PTCA (Figure 9).

All patients underwent acute and 7–10-day left ventriculography and coronary angiography. The immediate reduction of infarct vessel stenosis was apparent in the t-PA and PTCA randomized patients compared to t-PA alone (Figure 10). However, the 7-day patency was not significantly different between the two groups: 80% (12 of 15) for t-PA and PTCA versus 69% (9 of 13) for "t-PA only" therapy. Three of the "t-PA only" patients required crossover to PTCA for recurrent chest pain, electrocardiographic changes, and angiographically documented reocclusion at urgent repeat angiography.

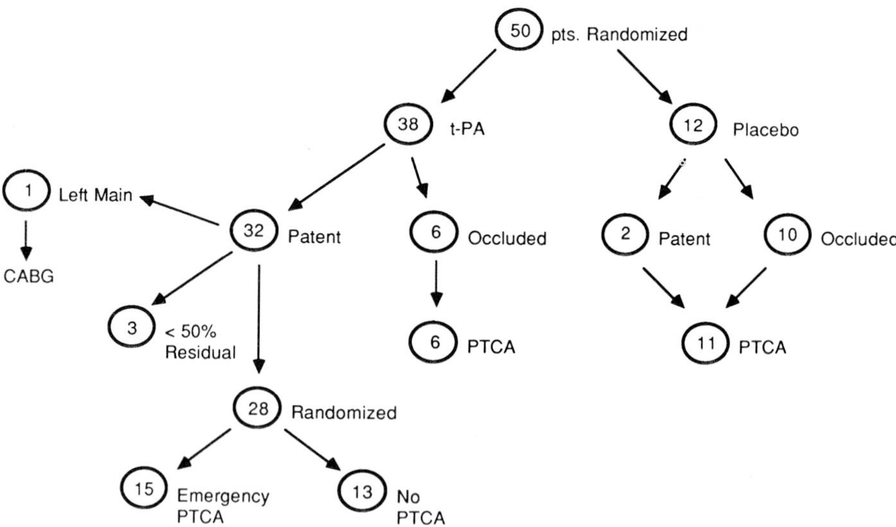

Figure 9   Flow chart of the 50 patients enrolled in a 3:1 randomized trial of intravenous t-PA versus placebo with a second randomization for patients with recanalization and suitable anatomy to emergency PTCA versus no PTCA. (From Ref. 37.)

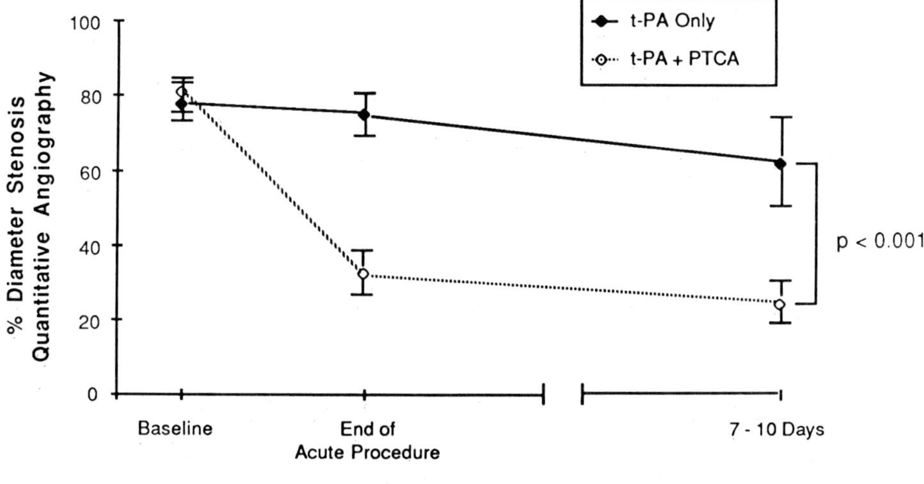

Figure 10   Percent diameter infarct vessel residual stenosis, as determined by quantitative coronary angiography for patients randomized to therapy with t-PA only versus t-PA and PTCA. Values are for those patients who manifested sustained patency throughout the 7- to 10-day study period. (From Ref. 37.)

Left ventricular function results for this trial are shown in Figure 11. Like the previous pilot study, t-PA and PTCA therapy—but not t-PA alone—augmented regional infarct-zone function. In this trial, the 15 patients who had PTCA as the primary method of recanalization showed significant infarct-zone functional recovery. This group included six patients who failed t-PA and nine placebo patients who exhibited persistent infarct-vessel occlusion.

A major revision of t-PA dosing was considered because early studies suggested that the reocclusion rate was high, ranging from 20–33% (21,22), despite concomitant heparin and antiplatelet therapy. At the Massachusetts General Hospital, Gold and colleagues found that reocclusion was occurring at times when the plasma t-PA level had fallen to levels below 1000 ng/ml (38). Using a low-dose, prolonged maintenance infusion, these investigators documented that: 1) angiographic residual stenosis decreased during the 6-hr infusion; 2) no significant further breakdown of fibrinogen occurred after the first hour of high-dose therapy; and 3) the incidence of reocclusion was reduced. This was an extremely important advance in t-PA pharmacology,

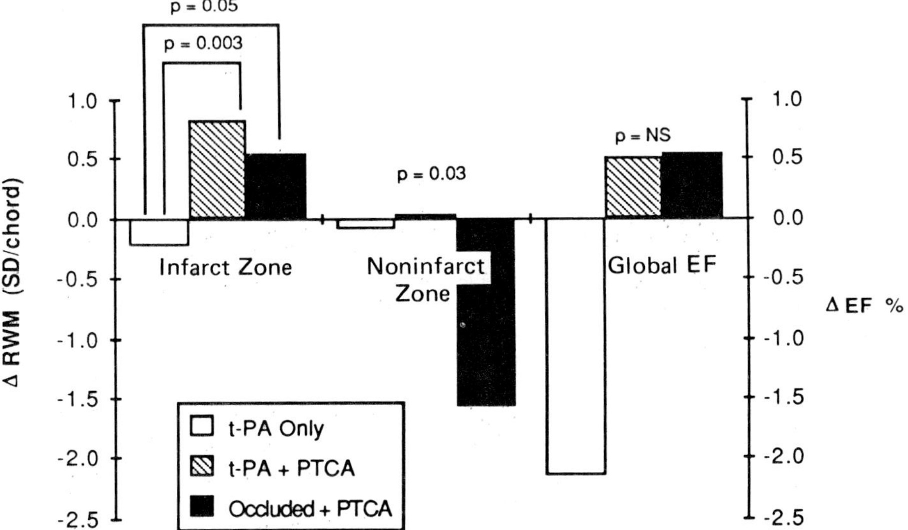

Figure 11   The change, from admission to day 7, in regional and global left ventricular function results for patients randomized to t-PA only, t-PA and PTCA, and patients who underwent PTCA as a primary method to achieve recanlization (after initially receiving placebo or experiencing failure of t-PA). Only patients who received PTCA therapy manifested a significant improvement of regional infarct-zone wall motion, expressed as standard deviation units per chord. Patients with an occluded infarct vessel were the only group exhibiting significant regression of the initial hyperkinesis of the noninfarct zone on admission ventriculography. None of the groups showed significant improvement in global ejection fraction. (From Ref. 37.)

because it set up the potential to defer definitive revascularization of the infarct vessel. The stage was set for larger trials to evaluate the optimal role and timing of PTCA after t-PA therapy.

VIII.   t-PA AND PTCA: ONGOING RANDOMIZED TRIALS

Several multicenter randomized trials are presently under way to evaluate combined therapy. First, the National Heart, Lung and Blood Institute Phase 2 trial, known as TIMI (Thrombolysis in Myocardial Infarction) consists of two separate substudies, the designs for which are reviewed elsewhere in this volume. Second, our Thrombolysis and Angioplasty in Myocardial Infarction (TAMI) trial is nearing completion. In this trial, 350 patients will receive intravenous t-PA and undergo acute catheterization. A 90-min infarct vessel angiogram is obtained to triage the patients as follows: 1) patients who fail t-PA undergo PTCA; 2) patients who recanalize after t-PA with a significant (>50%) residual stenosis, and who are suitable for PTCA, are randomized to immediate or late (7-day) PTCA; 3) patients with <50% residual stenosis are treated medically; and 4) patients with left main or equivalent anatomy undergo urgent surgical revascularization (Figure 12). Third, in the European Cooperative Study patients are randomized to either intravenous t-PA alone without catheterization or an aggressive arm of combined t-PA and PTCA. Its major endpoint is mortality. Fourth, the Johns Hopkins Medical Center is

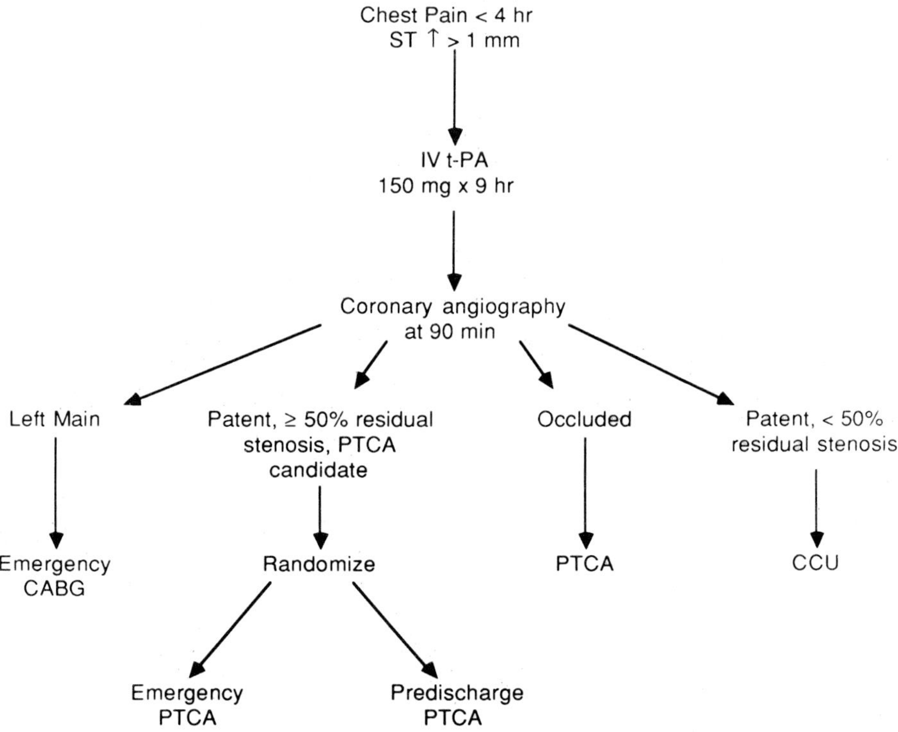

Figure 12   The Thrombolysis and Angioplasty in Myocardial Infarction (TAMI) Study design.

completing an approximately 200-patient, three-hospital trial of randomized, double-blind, intravenous placebo or t-PA therapy and a second randomization to PTCA on the third hospital day for all patients who demonstrated a patent infarct vessel during the acute catheterization.

IX. COMBINING t-PA AND PTCA: TIMING AND APPROACH

Cumulatively, these four studies will provide vital data on the optimal methods of combining t-PA-mediated thrombolysis and PTCA. Several important alternative strategies after intravenous t-PA therapy will be evaluated, including the following: 1) emergency PTCA, 2) deferred PTCA, 3) PTCA as needed, and 4) no PTCA. Each strategy has its distinct merits and disadvantages, as represented in Table 3. The recanalization rate would be expected to be the highest with emergency PTCA. This alternative provides for balloon dilation of the infarct vessel that has failed pharmacological therapy. The patients in the failed t-PA group, approximately 25% of patients treated, are a key subset who may benefit from aggressive, urgent PTCA. Unfortunately, there is no available clinical or noninvasive test that allows us to accurately diagnose which patients have reperfused after t-PA. The early catheterization provides the recanalization status and complete coronary anatomical information, identifying patients who appear to be at especially high risk, including

Table 3   Timing of PTCA

	Emergency	Deferred	As needed	No cath/PTCA
Recanalization rate	Potentially maximal	Intermediate	Reduced	Least
Initial recanalization status	Yes	No	No	No
Applicability	Least	Wide	Wide	Maximal
PTCA safety	?	May be improved	?	—
Bleeding complications	Maximum	Intermediate	Low	Minimal
Myocardial preservation/ mortality	?	?	?	?
Cost	Maximum	Intermediate	Reduced	Minimum

those with critical left main stenosis or advanced, severe three-vessel coronary artery disease. However, this strategy has obvious limited applicability. In addition, residual thrombus and activated platelets at or near the culprit coronary artery plaque may produce an increased risk associated with emergency PTCA compared to deferring the procedure until more complete dissolution of fibrin has occurred and antiplatelet therapy has taken effect. Beyond the unproven safety of emergency PTCA therapy of the coronary artery, a heightened risk of bleeding complications, particularly periaccess, would be anticipated because of invasive punctures while patients are receiving high-dose t-PA and heparin.

By deferring PTCA, several important advantages may be realized. First, the safety of the procedure may be increased, both in dilating the coronary artery and obtaining arterial access without concomitant fibrinolytic therapy. Second, this strategy is readily transferable to the community hospital not equipped with a cardiac catheterization and angioplasty facility. (Some patients may deteriorate before transfer arrangements are made, due to re-occlusion or extensive myocardial necrosis, and emergency PTCA or bypass surgery might be required.) Further, some patients may have more complete resolution of residual thrombus over 2 to 3 days and the overall need for PTCA might be reduced. Since this strategy does not allow for dilation of infarct vessels that fail t-PA, or those that reocclude prior to the deferred procedure, the actual number of PTCAs performed would be lessened by at least 25–30%, although this may be at the expense of reduced myocardial preservation and increased mortality compared to the aggressive emergency PTCA alternative.

The PRN (''as needed'') PTCA strategy would call for this procedure only if there was evidence of postinfarction ischemia or if an exercise test suggested reversible ischemia in the periinfarct zone. Although this strategy would provide considerably less anatomical or recanalization information, it has wide applicability and presumably lower costs. This type of strategy obligates recurrent myocardial ischemia, with overt expression of jeopardized, ''salvageable'' tissue, before intervention.

The ''t-PA only'' strategy would be the most widely applicable, require the smallest cost compared to other arms that incorporate PTCA, and would, by itself, be expected to reduce mortality compared to that of conventionally treated patients, as inferred from the Italian trial results.

X. PTCA: SUBSET ANALYSIS

Several key assumptions are inherent in the above approaches. First, several studies of myocardial reperfusion therapy have demonstrated the fundamental importance of early initiation (15,39). Second, approximately 10% of patients who receive t-PA therapy do not have a significant residual (>50% diameter reduction) atherosclerotic lesion. In our experience, most of these patients are younger, and they may have an increased incidence of underlying coronary artery spasm with only minimal intimal disease. Third, although some patients appear to have a tight atheromatous lesion acutely, a small percentage (5–10%) improve substantially over 1 to 4 weeks (40). Such patients probably have further dissolution of fibrin over time. Fourth, even with the remarkable advances in PTCA technology, there are some lesions and coronary artery anatomical subsets that cannot or should not be approached. This probably accounts for at least 10% of patients who recanalize after t-PA and will vary considerably among operators. In Figure 13, a hypothetical flow chart considers the outcome for 100 myocardial infarction patients treated with t-PA. If only patients who manifest recanalization after t-PA are considered for PTCA, only 40–50% of patients would be considered for PTCA. This figure

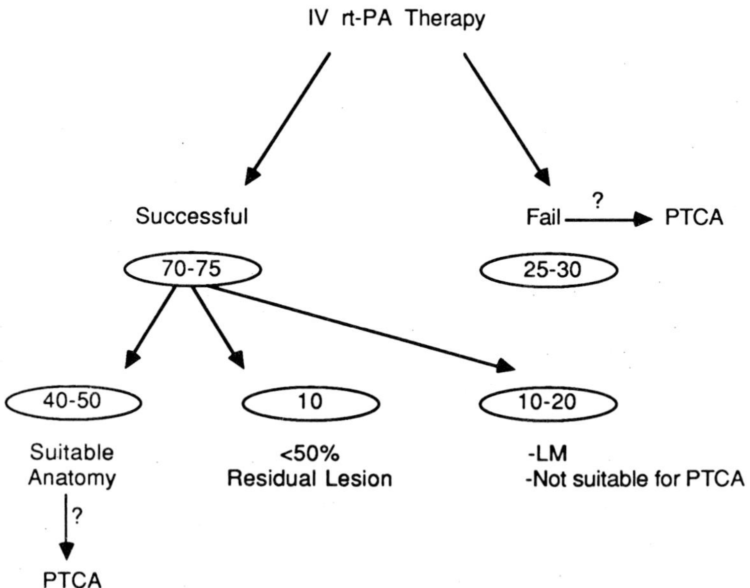

Figure 13   Hypothetical distribution of 100 patients receiving intravenous t-PA therapy for acute myocardial infarction. If PTCA is considered for patients who fail t-PA, an additional 20–30% of patients would be deemed suitable for this procedure. LM = critical left main or equivalent stenosis.

might go as high as 80% if ''failed t-PA'' patients receive PTCA on an emergency basis. Importantly, the combination of t-PA with PTCA is not for all patients, simply because some do not need it or their anatomy is not suitable.

In Table 4, patients and anatomical patterns are divided up into two groups: those who could derive potential benefit with PTCA after t-PA and those who could potentially be harmed. A very fundamental concept is that of ''high-risk'' subsets. These patients appear to be especially predisposed toward fatal or recurrent ischemic outcomes. This group includes patients with cardiogenic shock, who have approximately an 80% mortality without PTCA (41). Preliminary, nonrandomized studies suggest that PTCA may decrease the mortality for this subset to 40 or 50% (42–45). Patients with a proximal left anterior descending occlusion, with electrocardiographic ST-segment elevation across the precordial leads and in leads I and avL, have a poor prognosis with 20% in-hospital mortality (46) and significantly compromised left ventricular function in survivors. Definitive revascularization with PTCA or internal mammary artery grafting appears to be especially promising in this group of patients. We have noted a high mortality for patients with a proximal, hyperdominant right coronary artery occlusion. This is probably due to the extensive left ventricular necrosis overlying right ventricular infarction. Although our experience is relatively small and may be skewed, these patients appear prone to low-output syndrome, malignant arrhythmias, cardiac rupture, and fatal outcome. Similarly, patients with a prior transmural infarction, e.g., previous inferior and new anterior, have increased risk for power failure and death. Patients with an extremely tight residual stenosis (>95%, or less than 0.4 mm) are very prone to rethrombosis (47) and reinfarction and may derive benefit from mechanical dilation.

Table 4   PTCA After t-PA Therapy

Potential benefit	Potential harm
Failed t-PA therapy	Dissection-prone lesion/patient
High-risk subsets	lesion on bend
cardiogenic shock	diffuse disease
very high-grade residual stenosis	elderly
proximal left anterior descending	diabetes mellitus
? proximal, large RCA	''Low-risk'' anatomy
prior transmural infarction	Occluded contralateral vessel

There are, however, patient and anatomical groups that may be harmed by PTCA. Lesions that are prone to dissection include sites on a bend and those within an artery that contains diffuse, multilesion disease. Patients with diabetes mellitus or of advanced age also appear to be more prone to intimal dissection. In the setting of "low-risk" anatomy, defined as an infarct artery unlikely to spontaneously reocclude or one subserving a limited myocardial territory, PTCA may result in abrupt closure of not only the distal segment of the vessel, but the entire artery. This is quite uncommon but must be considered whenever dilation of such anatomy is contemplated. In the setting of chronically occluded contralateral vessel, loss of such an avenue for potential, recruitable collaterals leads to increased risk in the event of abrupt closure of the infarct vessel. This can result in precipitous hemodynamic collapse.

XI. PTCA: PITFALLS

Perhaps the major pitfall of PTCA in acute myocardial infarction is the potential for abrupt closure of the vessel. This may occur in a patient who is clinically and hemodynamically stable, with an electrocardiogram that has reverted to baseline and angiography that demonstrates a normal flow pattern. Such a patient may have had a partially or completely aborted myocardial infarction. In some cases, rather than ameliorating the residual stenosis, PTCA can result in a propagated intimal dissection and abrupt closure. Alternatively, the mechanical dilation and accompanying intimal denudation may result in recurrent thrombosis, possibly due to intense platelet activation. As in all cases of abrupt closure after PTCA, coronary vasospasm may also play a role.

The other major limitation of PTCA after t-PA is that patency at 7 to 10 days does not approach 100%. Our previous experience suggests that 10–20% of patients reocclude despite successful PTCA (30,37). This may be due to the same underlying mechanisms that result in acute failure. Reocclusion appears to occur in arteries without angiographic signs of even localized, minimal dissection. Recurrent thrombosis at the site of PTCA may account for the problem in most of these patients, but it has occurred despite heparin anticoagulation, antiplatelet therapy (aspirin and dipyridamole), and prolonged t-PA infusion. Perhaps the thrombotic tendency in some infarct vessels is so overwhelming that our current armamentarium cannot effectively combat the stimulus.

The incidence of restenosis—the major long-term complication of PTCA—in the setting of acute myocardial infarction is unknown. Preliminary studies suggest that it may be less than the 25–30% incidence after elective

PTCA (48). If this is confirmed in systematic long-term trials, fibrinolytic therapy may account for the apparent decrease in recurrence.

XII. FUTURE DIRECTIONS

Thrombolysis and angioplasty have emerged as a promising combination of pharmacological and mechanical therapy for acute myocardial infarction. Clearly, this is not a "fixed-dose" combination, as many patients would not need PTCA or could be detrimentally affected. Similarly, intravenous fibrinolytic treatment may not be appropriate in patients with high predisposition for bleeding.

The optimal timing of the PTCA is currently undergoing intense study. Although none of us would argue about the right time to administer fibrinolytic therapy—the earliest possible opportunity—there are many distinctive approaches for the timing of PTCA, as outlined above. As an outgrowth of the major ongoing randomized trials, high-risk and high-benefit subsets of patients will clearly be defined.

Significant limitations exist for both therapies. Intravenous t-PA leaves approximately 25% of infarct vessels with persistent occlusion, and a large percentage of these arteries have intraluminal thrombus. This enzyme is very potent, manifest by a coronary thrombolytic efficacy equivalent to intracoronary streptokinase, and by its potential for inducing bleeding.

Coronary angioplasty is relatively inaccessible and expensive. Although PTCA is accompanied by a high success rate, the procedure involves balloon trauma of acutely diseased intima and may result in either failure, abrupt closure, or subacute occlusion (at 1-week followup). Nonetheless, PTCA may be an extremely valuable method of establishing recanalization for those patients who fail thrombolytic therapy. In order to achieve maximal recovery of myocardial function, it may prove essential to perform PTCA early.

Adjunctive medical therapy with improved antiplatelet agents, including prostacyclin, heparinoids, and antiplatelet antibodies, will probably yield higher rates of long-term patency. As pharmacological advances with such therapy are made, the need for early, definitive revascularization will be reduced. Improved PTCA techniques, such as adjusting balloon length to that of the lesion and dual lumina to allow for continuous perfusion during balloon inflation, are already available and will continue to evolve. Better methods to address the underlying atherosclerotic plaque are also being developed, including mechanical stents for the vessel, introduced over a balloon catheter (49), atherectomy devices (50,51), and laser-balloon devices (52).

Further improvement with intravenous fibrinolytic therapy will also occur over the next few years, affording an even higher primary recanalization success rate. Ideally, an accurate, noninvasive marker will help us to identify patients who have not recanalized after plasminogen activator therapy, such that mechanical or intracoronary medical therapy could be applied as needed, without necessitating immediate cardiac catheterization in most patients.

In the early 1980s thrombolytic therapy and coronary angioplasty developed independently of, and in parallel with, the goal of coronary recanalization. Now these two therapies are being applied concurrently, and major clinical trials are addressing their optimal utilization. As results and experience continue to accrue, there will be considerable refinement in combining thrombolysis and angioplasty treatment for acute myocardial infarction.

REFERENCES

1. Gorlin R, Fuster V, Ambrose JA: Anatomic-physiologic links between acute coronary syndromes. Circulation 74:6–9, 1986.
2. Braunwald E: The aggressive treatment of acute myocardial infarction. Circulation 71:1087–1092, 1985.
3. Herrick JB: Clinical features of sudden obstruction of the coronary arteries. JAMA 59:2015–2020, 1912.
4. De Wood MA, Spores J, Notske R, Mouser LT, Bukrroughs R, Golden MS, Lang HT: Prevalence of total coronary occlusion during the early hours of transmural myocardial infarction. N Engl J Med 303:897, 1980.
5. Levin DC, Fallon JT: Significance of the angiographic morphology of localized coronary stenoses. Histopathologic correlations. Circulation 66:316, 1982.
6. Horie T, Sekiguchi M, Hirosawa K: Coronary thrombosis in pathogenesis of acute myocardial infarction. Histopathological study of coronary arteries in 108 necropsied cases using serial section. Br Heart J 40:1531, 1978.
7. Fuster V, Steele PM, Chesebro JH: Role of platelets and thrombosis in coronary atherosclerotic disease and sudden death. J Am Coll Cardiol 5:175B, 1985.
8. Davies MJ, Thomas A: Thrombosis and acute coronary artery lesions in sudden cardiac ischemic death. N Engl J Med 310:1137, 1984.
9. Falk E: Plaque rupture with severe pre-existing stenosis precipitating coronary thrombosis: characteristics of coronary atherosclerotic plaques underlying fatal occlusive thrombi. Br Heart J 50:127, 1983.
10. Roberts WC: Coronary arteries in fatal acute myocardial infarction. Circulation 45:215, 1972.
11. Reimer KA, Lowe JE, Rasmussen MM, Jennings RB: The wavefront phenomenon of ischemic cell death. I. Myocardial infarct size vs. duration of coronary occlusion in dogs. Circulation 56:786–794, 1977.

12. Rentrop KP: Thrombolytic therapy in patients with acute myocardial infarction. Circulation 71:627–631, 1985.

13. Kennedy JW, Ritchie JL, Davis KB, Stadius ML, Maynard C, Fritz JK: The western Washington randomized trial of intracoronary streptokinase in acute myocardial infarction. N Engl J Med 312:1073–1078, 1985.

14. Khaja F, Walton JA Jr, Brymer JF, Lo E, Osterberger L, O'Neill WW, Colfer HT, Weiss R, Lee T, Kurian T, Goldberg AD, Pitt B, Goldstein S: Intracoronary fibrinolytic therapy in acute myocardial infarction. N Engl J Med 308:1305–1311, 1983.

15. Gruppo Italiano Per Lo Studio Della Streptochinasi Nell'Infarcto Miocardio (GISSI): Effectiveness of intravenous thrombolytic treatment in acute myocardial infarction. Lancet 1:397–401, 1986.

16. Simoons ML, Brand M V/D, de Zwaan C, Verheugt FWA, Remme WJ, Serruys PW, Bar F, Res J, Krauss XH, Vermeer F: Improved survival after early thrombolysis in acute myocardial infarction. Lancet 2:578–582, 1985.

17. Laffel GL, Braunwald E: Thrombolytic therapy: a new strategy for the treatment of acute myocardial infarction. N Engl J Med 311:710–717, 770–776, 1984.

18. Collen D, Topol EJ, Tiefenbrunn AJ, Gold HK, Weisfeldt ML, Sobel BE, Leinbach RC, Brinker JA, Ludbrook PA, Yasuda I, Bulkley BH, Robison AK, Hutter AM, Bell WR, Spadaro JJ, Khaw BA, Grossbard EB: Coronary thrombosis with recombinant human tissue-type plasminogen activator: a prospective, randomized, placebo-controlled trial. Circulation 70:1012–1017, 1984.

19. Verstraete M, Bory M, Collen D, Erbel R, Lennane RJ, Mathey D, Michels HR, Schartl M, Uebis R, Bernard R, Brower RW, de Bono DP, Huhmann W, Lubsen J, Meyer J, Rutsch W, Schmidt W, von Essen R: Randomized trial of intravenous recombinant tissue-type plasminogen activator versus intravenous streptokinase in acute myocardial infarction. Lancet 1:842–847, 1985.

20. Van de Werf F, Ludbrook PA, Bergmann SR, Tiefenbrunn AJ, Fox KAA, de Geest H, Verstraete M, Collen D, Sobel BE: Coronary thrombolysis with tissue-type plasminogen activator in patients with evolving myocardial infarction. N Engl J Med 310:609–613, 1984.

21. The TIMI Study Group: The thrombolysis in myocardial infarction (TIMI) trial. N Engl J Med 312:932–936, 1985.

22. Williams DO, Borer J, Braunwald E, Chesebro JH, Cohen LS, Dalen J, Dodge HT, Francis CK, Knatterud G, Ludbrook P, Markis JE, Mueller H, Desvigne-Nickens P, Passamani ER, Powers ER, Rao AK, Roberts R, Ross A, Ryan TJ, Sobel BE, Winniford M, Zaret B: Intravenous recombinant tissue-type plasminogen activator in patients with acute myocardial infarction: a report from the NHLBI thrombolysis in myocardial infarction trial. Circulation 73(2):338–346, 1986.

23. Swan HJC: Thrombolysis in acute myocardial infarction: treatment of the underlying coronary artery disease. Circulation 66(5):914–916, 1982.

24. Meyer J, Merx W, Schmitz H, Erbel R, Kiesslich T, Dorr R, Lambertz H, Bethge C, Krebs W, Bardos P, Minale C, Messmer BJ, Effert S: Percutaneous

transluminal coronary angioplasty immediately after intracoronary streptolysis of transmural myocardial infarction. Circulation 66(5):905–913, 1982.

25. Kitazume H, Iwama T, Suzuki A: Combined thrombolytic therapy and coronary angioplasty for acute myocardial infarction. Am Heart J 111:826–832, 1986.

26. Erbel R, Pop T, Meinertz T, Kasper W, Schreiner G, Henkel B, Henrichs KJ, Pfeiffer C, Rupprecht HJ, Meyer J: Combined medical and mechanical recanalization in acute myocardial infarction. Cathet Cardiovasc Diag 11:361–377, 1985.

27. Papapietro SE, MacLean WAH Jr, Stanley AWH, Hess RG, Corley N, Arciniegas JA, Cooper TB: Percutaneous transluminal coronary angioplasty after intracoronary streptokinase in evolving acute myocardial infarction. Am J Cardiol 55:48–53, 1985.

28. Kalbfleisch J, Friedman M, Slagle R, Brewer D, McEntee W, Roye A, Ross W, Hawkins H, Conrad L, Ong YS: A randomized trial of immediate coronary angioplasty following intracoronary thrombolysis in acute myocardial infarction. J Am Coll Cardiol 3(abstr):576, 1984.

29. O'Neill W, Timmis G, Bourdillon P, Lai P, Ganghadarhan V, Walton J, Ramos R, Laufer N, Gordon S, Schork MA, Pitt B: A prospective randomized clinical trial of intracoronary streptokinase versus coronary angioplasty therapy of acute myocardial infarction. N Engl J Med 314:814–828, 1986.

30. Timmis GC, O'Neill W, Bakalyar D, Lai PY, Gordon S: Effect of reperfusion adequacy on ventricular function versus infarction size. Circulation 72:III-308, 1985.

31. Diltz E, O'Neill W, Walton J, Bourdillon P, Laufer N, Nicklas J: Regional myocardial perfusion during medical revascularization in acute myocardial infarction. J Am Coll Cardiol 5:397, 1985.

32. Brown BG, Gallery CA, Badger RJ, Kennedy JW, Mathey D, Bolson EL, Dodge HT: Incomplete lysis of thrombus in the moderate underlying atherosclerotic lesion during intracoronary infusion of streptokinase for acute myocardial infarction: quantitative angiographic observations. Circulation 73:653–661, 1985.

33. Fung AY, Lai P, Juni JE, Bourdillon PD, Walton J, Laufer N, Buda A, Pitt B, O'Neill W: Prevention of subsequent exercise induced periinfarct ischemia by emergency coronary angioplasty in acute myocardial infarction: comparison with intracoronary streptokinase. J Am Coll Cardiol (in press, 1986).

34. Fung AY, Lai P, Topol EJ, Bates ER, Bourdillon PDV, Walton JA Jr, Mancini GBJ, Kryski T, Pitt B, O'Neill WW: Myocardial salvage by coronary angioplasty following thrombolytic failure in acute myocardial infarction. Am J Cardiol 59 (in press, 1986).

35. Topol EJ, Fung AY, Kline E, Kaplan L, Landis D, Strozeski M, Burney RE, Pitt B, O'Neill WW: Safety of helicopter transport and out-of-hospital intravenous fibrinolytic therapy in patients with evolving myocardial infarction. Cathet Cardiovasc Diag 12:151–155, 1986.

36. Topol EJ, Eha JE, Brin KP, Shapiro EP, Weiss JL, Riegel MB, Gottlieb SO,

Brinker JA: Applicability of percutaneous transluminal coronary angioplasty to patients with recombinant tissue plasminogen activator mediated thrombolysis. Cathet Cardiovasc 11:337–348, 1985.

37. Topol EJ, O'Neill WW, Walton JA, Bourdillon PDV, Bates ER, Langburd A, Baumann G, Burney RE, Kline E, Schork, MA, Pitt B: Preliminary report of a randomized, placebo controlled trial of recombinant tissue plasminogen activator and emergency coronary angioplasty in acute myocardial infarction. Circulation, 1987 (in press).

38. Gold HK, Leinbach RC, Garabedian HD, Yasuda T, Johns JA, Grossbard EB, Palacios I, Collen D: Acute coronary reocclusion after thrombolysis with recombinant human tissue-type plasminogen activator: prevention by a maintenance infusion. Circulation 73(2):347–352, 1986.

39. Mathey DG, Sheehan FH, Schofer J, Dodge HT: Time from onset of symptoms to thrombolytic therapy: a major determinant of myocardial salvage in patients with acute transluminal infarction. J Am Coll Cardiol 6:518–525, 1985.

40. Schmidt WG, Essen RR, Uebis R, Effert S, Rutsch W, Schartl M, Schmutzler H, Erbel R, Meyer J: Thrombolytic treatment of acute myocardial infarction with recombinant-tissue type plasminogen activator: coronary state after 4 weeks. J Am Coll Cardiol 7:16A, 1986.

41. Scheidt S, Wilner G, Mueller H, et al: Intraaortic balloon counter-pulsation in caridogenic shock. Report of a cooperative clinical trial. N Engl J Med 289:288–979, 1973.

42. O'Neill W, Erbel R, Laufer N, Walton J, Bates E, Topol E, Bourdillon PD, Meyer J, Pitt B: Coronary angioplasty therapy of cardiogenic shock complicating acute myocardial infarction. Circulation 72:III-309, 1985.

43. Brown TM Jr, Iannone LA, Gordon DF, Wickemeyer WJ, Wheeler WS, Rough RR: Percutaneous myocardial reperfusion (PMR) reduces mortality in acute myocardial infarction (MI) complicated by cardiogenic shock. Circulation 72: III-309, 1985.

44. Shani J, Rivera M, Greengart A, Hollander G, Kaplan P, Lichstein E: Percutaneous transluminal coronary angioplasty in cardiogenic shock. J Am Coll Cardiol 7:149A, 1986.

45. Rutherford BD, Hartzler GO, McConahay DR, Johnson WL Jr: Direct balloon angioplasty during acute myocardial infarction in patients with severely compromised hemodynamics. Circulation 72:III-308, 1985.

46. DeBusk RF, Blomqvist CG, Kouchoukos NT, Luepker RV, Miller HS, Moss AJ, Pollock ML, Reeves TJ, Selvester RH, Stason WB, Wagner GS, William VL: Identification and treatment of low-risk patients after acute myocardial infarction and coronary-artery bypass graft surgery. N Engl J Med 314:161–166, 1986.

47. Harrison DG, Ferguson DW, Collins SM, Skorton DJ, Ericksen EE, Kioschos M, Marcus ML, White CW: Rethrombosis after reperfusion with streptokinase: importance of geometry of residual lesions. Circulation 69(5):991–999, 1984.

48. Kander N, O'Neill WW, Topol E, Walton JA Jr, Bourdillon PD, Bates E,

Kryski T, Pitt B: Prognosis after acute coronary angioplasty therapy of acute myocardial infarction. J Am Coll Cardiol 7:150A, 1986.

49. Palmaz JC, Sibbitt RR, Tio FO, Reuter SR, Peters JE, Garcia F: Expandable intraluminal vascular graft: a feasibility study. Surgery 99:199–205, 1986.

50. Lai P, O'Neill WW, Auth D, Abrams GD, Glass H, Long R, Pitt B: Nonsurgical human coronary endarterectomy: use of a mechanical rotary catheter. Circulation 72:III-371, 1985.

51. Simpson JB, Johnson DE, Thapliyal HV, Marks DS, Braden LJ: Transluminal atherectomy: a new approach to the treatment of atherosclerotic vascular disease. Circulation 72:III-146, 1985.

52. Sanborn TA, Sinclair IN, Serur JR, Spokojny AM, Bourgelais D, Schoen FJ, Faxon DP, Ryan TJ, Spears JR: In vivo laser thermal seal of neointimal dissection after balloon angioplasty in rabbit atherosclerosis. Circulation 72:III-469, 1985.

7

Prevention of Acute Reocclusion After Thrombolysis with Intravenous Recombinant Tissue Plasminogen Activator

Herman K. Gold and Robert C. Leinbach
*Massachusetts General Hospital
and Harvard Medical School
Boston, Massachusetts*

I. INTRODUCTION

Intravenous recombinant human tissue-type plasminogen activator (rt-PA) given within 6 hr of the onset of transmural myocardial infarction produces satisfactory reflow in 60–85% (1–3) of patients. However, in the early studies, coronary reocclusion occurred within 1 hr to 10 days in 20–45% of patients (1,4,5), a reocclusion rate that is equal to or higher than that previously reported with streptokinase (range 5–29%) and possibly related to the same features that make rt-PA a desirable thrombolytic agent, i.e., clot specificity and short half-life.

The list of variables that could affect coronary reocclusion includes: 1) severity of residual coronary stenosis, 2) persistence of intraluminal thrombus, 3) inadequate heparin anticoagulation, and 4) cumulative dose of rt-PA and duration of infusion. Two preparations of rt-PA were studied, with half-lives of 4.1 and 5.5 min, respectively (6).

II. INITIAL EXPERIENCE WITH rt-PA

The initial studies (1–3) of rt-PA utilized a predominantly (>95%) two-chain rt-PA produced on a small scale at Genentech, Inc. (product code G11021).

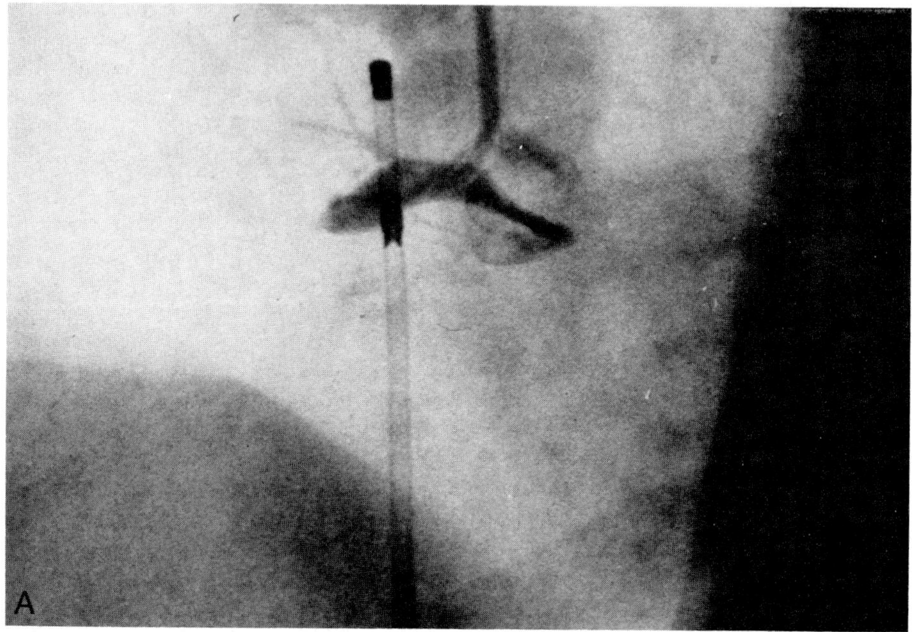

Figure 1   Angiographic frames from a patient with proximal right coronary artery occlusion (A) before intravenous rt-PA (LAO view), (B) after rt-PA (RAO view), and (C) 21 min after cessation of rt-PA (LAO view). The site of reocclusion appears to be at the point of maximal stenosis.

These studies [with intravenous rt-PA (G11021)] were begun in patients with acute coronary occlusion under angiographic control. The selection criteria were: 1) age less than 70 years, 2) chest pain of less than 6 hr duration, 3) ST elevation equal to or greater than 0.1 mV in two standard leads, and 4) no contraindication to thrombolytic therapy. rt-PA was not administered until angiographic demonstration of complete coronary occlusion.

The dose was 0.4 to 0.75 mg/kg given over 60–120 min. Angiography was repeated at 15–30 min intervals with a primary endpoint at 90 min and repeat angiography 1 hr after cessation of rt-PA infusion. In the initial studies of 13 patients, intravenous rt-PA produced reflow within 90 min in 11 (85%). Reflow was defined as complete antegrade filling of the obstructed coronary artery with washout within four or five cardiac cycles. Heparin was given at the beginning of the catheterization in a 5000-U bolus followed by a contin-

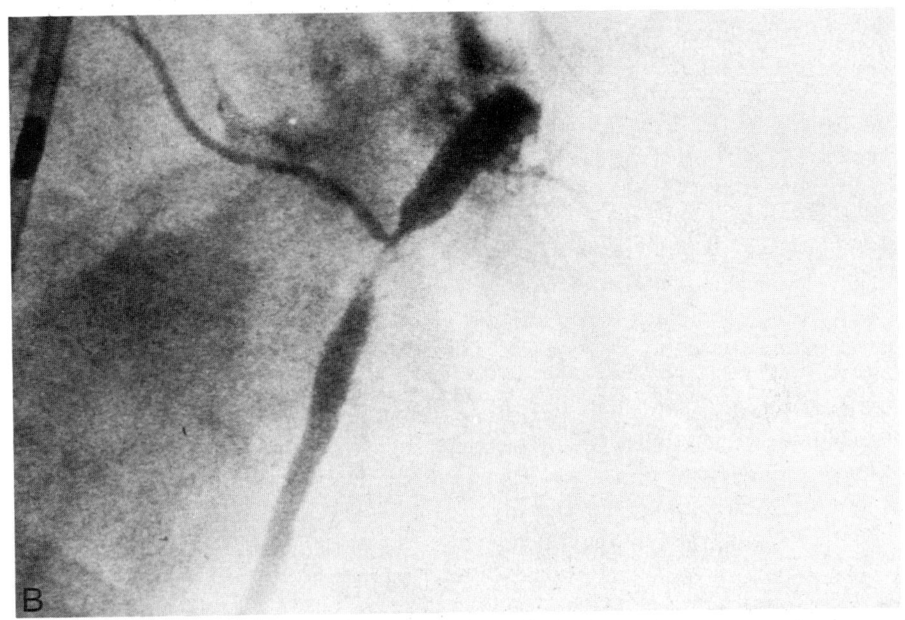

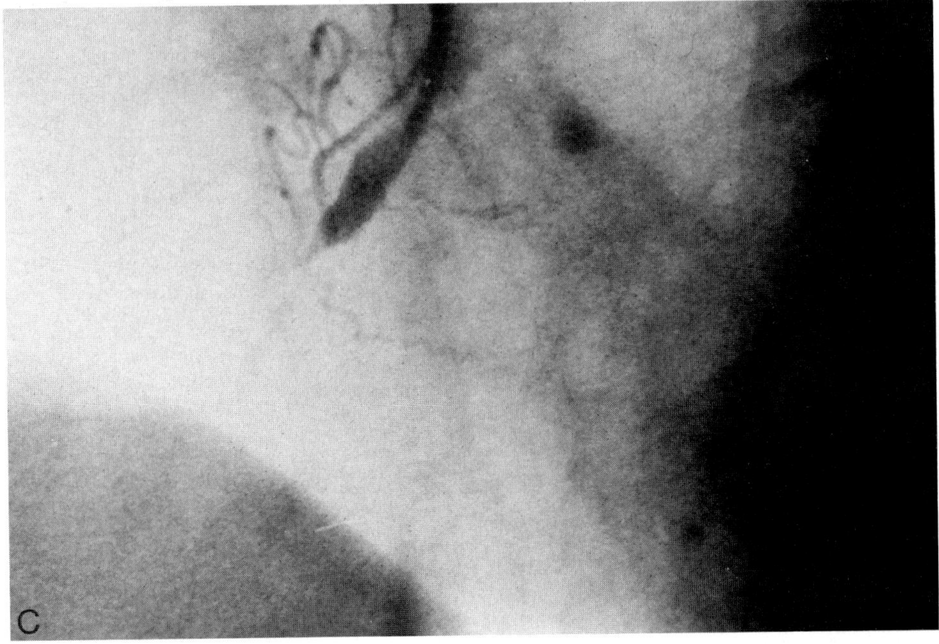

uous intravenous infusion of 1000 U/hr. No antiplatelet drugs were used. All patients also received a continuous infusion of intravenous nitroglycerin in a dose designed to reduce systolic arterial pressure by 10%.

Despite maintenance heparin and nitroglycerin, five of the 11 reflowed cases (45%) showed coronary reocclusion during the 60-min post-rt-PA observation period. Figure 1 illustrates the problem. In this patient, reflow was documented after 46 min of rt-PA, and reocclusion occurred 21 min after its cessation.

Clinical and angiographic characteristics of the 11 patients with reflow were further evaluated in a search for causes of reocclusion. Comparing the five patients reoccluding with the six showing stable reflow, no difference was found with respect to age, sex, vessel involved, time to reflow, or rt-PA dose. A highly significant difference was found in residual stenosis at 90 min quantitatively measured by the technique of Brown et al. (7). Table 1 lists angiographic findings and reocclusion times in these 11 patients. Residual coronary stenosis averaged $87 \pm 2\%$ and residual lumen diameter 0.37 ± 0.1 mm in the patients reoccluding, compared to $69 \pm 8\%$ and 0.85 ± 0.2 mm in the patients with stable reflow. Both differences were significant at the 0.01 level. Filling defects were seen in both groups.

Plasma rt-PA levels measured in the five patients showing reocclusion

Table 1   Coronary Reocclusion After rt-PA

	Patient	Percent stenosis	Diameter (mm)	Filling defect	Time to reocclusion (min)
Group A	1	85	0.43	−	31
	2	87	0.36	−	48
	3	85	0.44	+	21
	4	88	0.28	−	60
	5	90	0.34	−	24
Group B	6	58	0.91	−	—
	7	67	1.1	+	—
	8	75	0.64	−	—
	9	76	0.75	−	—
	10	66	0.77	−	—
	11	69	0.98	+	—
p value (A vs. B)		<0.01	<0.01		

are shown in Figure 2. Reocclusion developed when the blood level fell to 25% of the steady-state level measured just prior to the termination of infusion or to an average level of 0.35 μg/ml, always within 60 min of cessation of infusion.

Analysis of hemostatic parameters during rt-PA infusion also failed to identify patients destined to reocclude. No differences were found in total fibrinogen, plasminogen, α_2-antiplasmin, partial thromboplastin time (PTT), or plasma rt-PA levels. Fibrinogen levels measured by the Ratnoff and Menzie method fell to an average of 78% of control; PTT was always greater than 100 s prior to and at the time of reocclusion; plasminogen fell to 30% of control; and α_2-antiplasmin fell to 70% of control. Disappearance curves for rt-PA (G11021) showed that clearance is biexponential with half-lives of 5.5 and 45 min. Reocclusion therefore occurred after about seven rapid-phase half-lives.

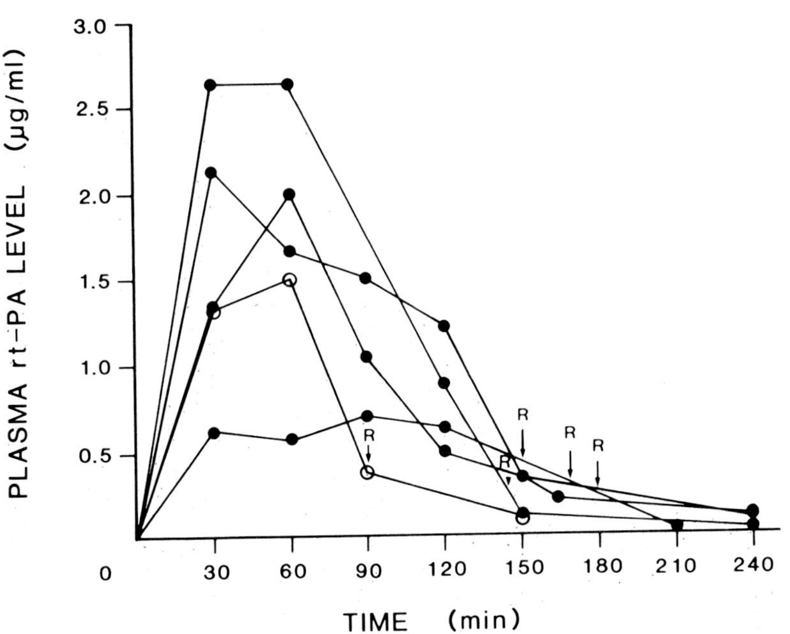

Figure 2 A plot of plasma rt-PA level against time in five patients showing coronary reocclusion after cessation of rt-PA infusion. The duration of the infusion is indicated by the closed and open circles and the point of reocclusion marked by the letter R.

III. ANIMAL STUDIES OF RESIDUAL CORONARY STENOSIS AND REOCCLUSION

To analyze the pathology of reocclusion and to compare reocclusion frequency after administration of rt-PA, streptokinase, and urokinase, we turned to a canine model. Left anterior descending (LAD) thrombosis was induced below the major diagonal branch using a local installation of blood and thrombin into a temporarily isolated segment previously traumatized by external compression with forceps. A 1-cm stable clot was reliably induced. After LAD thrombosis for 30 min, intravenous rt-PA given at 15 μg/kg/min produced uniform reflow after 28 $\pm$ 13 min. Intravenous streptokinase at 625 U/kg/min and intravenous urokinase at 1000 U/kg/min for 30 min followed by intracoronary urokinase at 1000 U/kg/min for 30 min (if necessary) also produced reflow in all preparations at 34 $\pm$ 24 and 65 $\pm$ 23 min, respectively. Reocclusion was not seen.

Further canine experiments were performed with the addition of a high-grade external stenosis adjusted to reduce resting coronary blood flow to 40% of normal, which angiographically is approximately 80% diameter stenosis. This stenosis was placed within the clotted segment.

The effect of the external stenosis on reflow rate following the previously described doses of rt-PA, streptokinase, and urokinase is shown in Table 2. The reflow rate was reduced to 33% (2/6) with streptokinase and to 50% (3/6) with urokinase. In contrast, the ability of rt-PA to produce reflow was not altered or significantly delayed. However, all animals showed coronary reocclusion with a 60-min postinfusion observation period. In all cases the reocclusion occurred at the point of maximal stenosis. Pathological sections at this site (Figure 3) revealed compression of the artery, widespread endothelial loss, and occlusion by platelet-rich fibrin thrombi. Such thrombi

Table 2   Thrombolysis in Stenotic Model

	SK	UK	rt-PA
Number of dogs	6	6	6
Number with reflow	2	3	8
Time to reflow (min)	59	40 $\pm$ 10	27 $\pm$ 10
Number with reocclusion	2	3	8

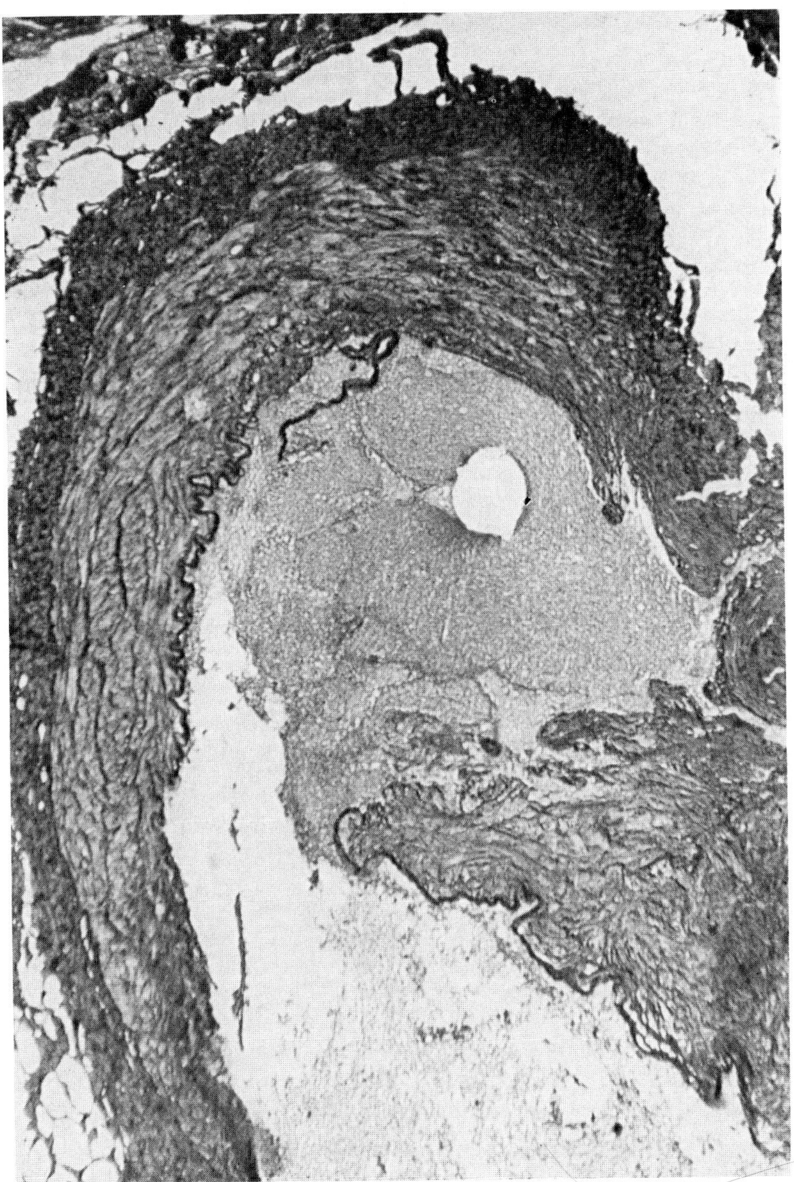

Figure 3   A section taken from the point of maximal stenosis in the canine model after coronary reocclusion. Disruption of the intima and internal elastic lamina is apparent with overlying platelet fibrin thrombus. The thrombus in vivo was completely occlusive.

were seen even when systemic fibrinogen levels had fallen to less than 10 mg/dl (urokinase dogs).

We concluded that the probable mechanism of reocclusion in patients with high-grade residual stenosis was primarily thrombotic and that reocclusion could not be reliably prevented by therapeutic levels of heparin anticoagulation or high doses of short-term thrombolytic agents.

IV. MANAGEMENT OF REOCCLUSION

Treatment of reocclusion is often unsatisfactory. Retreatment of a patient with intravenous rt-PA may require infusions of 30–45 min at doses equal to or greater than the previous thrombolytic dose to reestablish antegrade coronary flow. We have encountered this delay despite retreatment soon after the acute onset of recurrent injury. Moreover, administration of rt-PA in a second thrombolytic dose may be associated with a significant depression of systemic fibrinogen. Emergency percutaneous transluminal coronary angioplasty (PTCA) requires instrumentation and catheterization with delays not well tolerated by repeatedly ischemic myocardium. Prevention of reocclusion is the preferable approach.

The interrelationship between residual stenosis and reocclusion and the demonstration that reocclusion is thrombotic involving both platelets and fibrin suggests several preventive measures. Urgent PTCA is successful in above 80% of cases (8,9), reducing stenosis to a level less than that seen in patients with stable reflow (Table 1). However, in-hospital reocclusion is seen at a rate higher than the rate after elective PTCA and, more importantly, this approach commits patients to acute angiography since the prediction of acute reocclusion depends on the angiographic appearance of the residual coronary lesion. Also, part of this residual stenosis may be mural thrombus or other reversible occlusion since angiography after 1 week often shows further improvement in percent stenosis.

Antiplatelet agents have been tried in streptokinase-treated patients, but reocclusion has not been prevented (10). It is possible that more potent and more readily reversible antiplatelet agents will be developed and may be effective. However, the present anticoagulation program may have to be modified since a combination of fibrinolysis, heparin anticoagulation, and a potent platelet-blocking drug may not be clinically tolerated, although some investigators report success with intensive heparin anticoagulation (11).

The fibrin that is laid down despite anticoagulation in areas of high-grade stenosis may evolve from circulating fibrinogen after withdrawal of rt-PA or from platelets activated at the stenotic injured site which are capable of

Table 3   Plasma Levels of rt-PA[a] at
Different Infusion Rates

Dose mg/kg/90 min	n	Steady-state plasma rt-PA levels (μg/ml)
0.3–0.39	6	0.52 ± 0.15
0.4–0.47	7	0.76 ± 0.29
0.5	8	0.83 ± 0.19
0.625	18	

[a]Product number G11021.

adhering and aggregating despite systemic fibrinogenolysis. Since this is a dynamic process it is plausible that this platelet-fibrin plug could be prevented by maintenance of adequate levels of a thrombolytic agent (12). To accomplish this without severe systemic fibrinogenolysis, it is necessary to use a relatively clot-specific agent.

The average plasma level of rt-PA at which reocclusion reoccurred in the setting of high-grade stenosis was known (Figure 2; 0.35 μg/ml). We also knew the dose of rt-PA capable of producing levels higher than this. Table 3 demonstrates plasma levels in patients at four dose ranges. From these data and disappearance curves, we calculated that a dose of 0.5 mg/kg given over 4 hr would produce plasma rt-PA levels higher than those associated with reocclusion. The likelihood of further systemic fibrinogen breakdown and depletion of other coagulation factors was uncertain.

V. EFFECT OF A MAINTENANCE rt-PA INFUSION

In a second group of 16 patients, rt-PA (G11021) was again given with 13 (81%) showing reflow at 90 min. Seven of these 13 patients showed residual coronary stenosis estimated from video playback to be 80% or greater. These seven patients received a 4-hr maintenance infusion of rt-PA of 0.5 mg/kg in addition to uninterrupted heparin anticoagulation.

Reocclusion was judged angiographically 1 hr into the maintenance infusion and at repeat angiography at 10–14 days. Serial levels of plasma rt-PA, fibrinogen, plasminogen, and α_2-antiplasmin were followed. The quantitative angiographic results of these 13 cases are given in Table 4.

Table 4   Coronary Reocclusion and rt-PA Maintenance

	Patient	rt-PA maintenance	Percent stenosis	Diameter (mm)	Filling defect	Time to reocclusion (days)
Group C	1	Y	91	0.34	+	—
	2	Y	86	0.54	+	—
	3	Y	82	0.68	+	7
	4	Y	84	0.51	−	—
	5	Y	78	0.83	+	—
	6	Y	82	0.54	+	—
	7	Y	86	0.44	−	—
Group D	8	N	53	1.27	−	—
	9	N	46	1.3	−	—
	10	N	66	0.9	+	—
	11	N	65	1.02	+	—
	12	N	78	0.42	−	—
	13	N	72	0.89	+	10

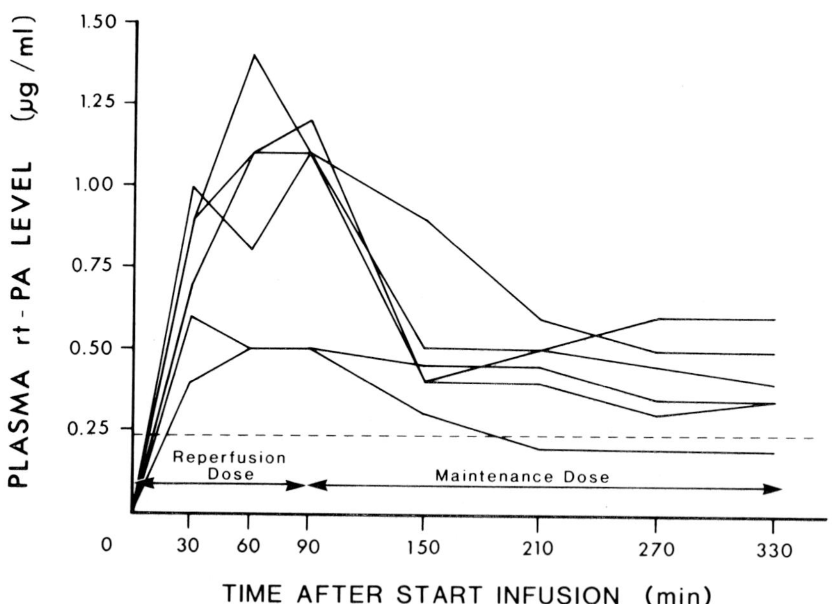

Figure 4   Plasma rt-PA levels in six patients treated with a 4-hr maintenance infusion of 0.5 mg/kg beginning at the 90-min point immediately after cessation of the thrombolytic dose. The average maintenance level was 0.38 μg/ml.

No patient with high-grade residual stenosis showed reocclusion within 1 hr of cessation of rt-PA. Angiography at 10–14 days showed persistent patency in six of seven. At the 90-min point of rt-PA infusion the mean percent stenosis and luminal diameter for these seven patients was 84 ± 4% and 0.55 ± 0.16 mm, compared to 84 ± 2% and 0.37 ± 0.1 mm in the previous group with 100% acute reocclusion (Table 1). One patient in the group with less than 80% stenosis showed later reocclusion.

Plasma levels of rt-PA obtained by the 4-hr infusion of 0.5 mg/kg are shown for six of the seven patients with high-grade stenosis in Figure 4. The average maintenance level of 0.38 ± 0.12 µg/ml, with only one patient falling below 0.25 µg/ml. This infusion resulted in moderate additional decreases in plasma fibrinogen falling to 62% of control (Figure 5). The additional fall in plasminogen and α_2-antiplasmin was slight.

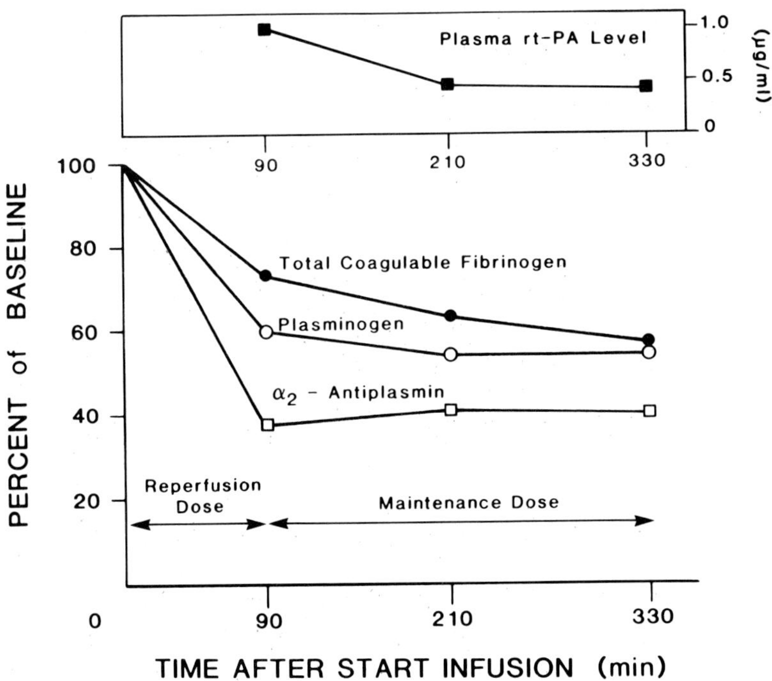

Figure 5   Total coagulable fibrinogen, plasminogen, and α_2-antiplasmin are shown as percent of baseline during the 90-min thrombolytic infusion (reperfusion dose) and the 4-hr maintenance. The mean plasma rt-PA level is shown above.

VI. STUDIES WITH rt-PA (G11035)

In 1985 a change in production methods at Genentech, Inc., led to the generation of rt-PA in a predominantly (60–80%) single-chain form (G11035). We tested the thrombolytic potency and the pharmacokinetics of this new form in 23 additional patients and compared responses to previous rt-PA (G11021) infusions in 40 patients (Table 5). An infusion of 9.4 μg/kg/min of rt-PA (G11035) was required to produce steady-state plasma levels equivalent to doses of 7 μg/kg/min of rt-PA (G11021) with equivalent thrombolytic potency. The rapid phase half-life was found to be shorter with rt-PA (G11035) (4.1 min compared to 5.5 min with G11021).

At the dose of 9.4 μg/kg/min, rt-PA (G11035) caused minimal fibrinogen degeneration, but the time required to achieve reflow averaged 60 ± 26 min. Therefore, we advanced the dose to 11 μg/kg/min with fibrinogen levels maintained at 71 ± 5% of control. This dose is equivalent to 1 mg/kg given over 90 min.

After administration of 1 mg/kg of rt-PA (G11035) over 90 min, we identified 22 patients with residual coronary stenosis of 80% or more and administered a maintenance rt-PA infusion (0.8 mg/kg/4 hr) in 12. Ten randomly selected patients with similar residual coronary stenosis served as controls. The results are shown in Table 6. A maintenance infusion of 0.8 mg/kg/4 hr of rt-PA (G11035) produced maintenance blood levels of 0.72 ± 0.5 μg/ml and was associated with no in-hospital reocclusions. A remarkable additional finding was that even without a maintenance rt-PA infusion, the reocclusion rate in patients who had received 1 mg/kg/90 min was only two

Table 5   Comparison of G11021 and G11035

	Dose μg/kg/min	n	Percent reflow	Time to reflow (min)	Residual filling defect	Fibrinogen percent of control	Plasma level rt-PA (μg/ml)
rt-PA	4	6	0	—	—	75 ± 3[a]	0.52 ± 0.15[b]
G11021	5.3	16	81	63 ± 19[b]	8/12	69 ± 10	0.81 ± 0.22
	7	18	83	55 ± 19	3/15	53 ± 12	1.1 ± 0.18
G11035	7	5	40	82 ± 11	2/2	94 ± 6	0.7 ± 0.14
	9.4	7	86	60 ± 25	2/6	85 ± 12	1.3 ± 0.45
	11	11	82	48 ± 17	2/9	68 ± 4	1.8 ± 0.4

[a]SE.
[b]SD.

Table 6   Reocclusion After rt-PA G11035

n	Lytic dose (mg/kg/90 min)	Maintenance dose (mg/kg/24 hr)	Stenosis at 90 min (%)	Follow-up stenosis (%)	Maintenance rt-PA level (μg/ml)	Reoc-clusion (%)
10	1.0	0	82.5 ± 4.6	83 ± 11.6	—	20
12	1.0	0.8	83.0 ± 4.5	70 ± 12.2	0.70 ± 0.5	0

[a] $p < 0.05$ compared to stenosis at 90 min.

out of 10 (20%). However, reduction in late coronary stenosis was seen only with rt-PA maintenance (83 ± 4.5% to 70 ± 12.2%; $p < 0.05$), and recurrent ischemia was seen in six of the 10 patients not receiving rt-PA maintenance. Angina developed in only one of 10 rt-PA maintenance patients (Table 7).

This experience with rt-PA suggests that a 4-hr maintenance dose is effective in preventing reocclusion, and also that infusion at 1 mg/kg given for the standard 90-min thrombolytic period without maintenance produces changes capable of preventing reocclusion despite high-grade residual coronary stenosis. The nature of these changes is not yet defined. Possibly residual mural thrombus is more effectively cleared, and possibly undefined hemostatic parameters are altered for a time longer than the rt-PA half-life. Nevertheless, the prevention of reocclusion without maintenance rt-PA appears tenuous, with recurrent ischemia frequent in this group and no significant reduction in coronary stenosis by hospital discharge. In contrast, residual ischemia is rare after rt-PA maintenance, and residual stenosis frequently falls to less critical levels.

Table 7   In-Hospital Ischemic Events and rt-PA Maintenance

	Maintenance (12)	No maintenance (10)
Rest ischemia	1	6
Silent reocclusion	0	2
Myocardial infarction	0	0
Total	1 (8%)	8 (80%)

$p < 0.002$.

VII. FUTURE DIRECTIONS

It is generally agreed that rapid thrombolysis is the treatment of choice for transmural myocardial infarction (13). Experience with various reflow techniques has shown that the most rapid thrombolysis for patients experiencing myocardial infarction out of hospital is by intravenous pharmacological methods (14). The reflow rate with intravenous rt-PA in our experience exceeds 80% within 90 min. Therefore, a technique is available for thrombolysis without complicated instrumentation which does not produce severe systemic fibrinogen depletion.

Further, it is possible to prevent reocclusion for more than 1 week by heparin anticoagulation and an uninterrupted crossover from thrombolytic rt-PA doses to a 4-hr maintenance infusion. Fibrinogen depletion remains moderate even after the 4-hr maintenance. Therefore, one can treat patients with transmural myocardial infarction with rt-PA and achieve a high reflow rate and subsequently prevent reocclusion without acute myocardial intervention. Since approximately 60% of patients will have high-grade residual coronary stenosis after initial thrombolysis, one would predict that a uniform policy of maintenance rt-PA infusion would mean overtreatment of some patients. Nevertheless, most patients could be spared emergency angiography. PTCA and bypass surgery could be delayed until the demonstration of recurrent ischemia either spontaneously or during stress.

A reduction in early instrumentation would result in a marked diminution in bleeding problems, and a delay in PTCA may lead to a higher ultimate success rate and a lower frequency of post-PTCA reocclusion. The overall PTCA and coronary bypass requirements may be reduced by more complete resolution of coronary obstruction. This approach is also well suited for future developments in thrombolytic agents. A third-generation rt-PA may prove even more effective primarily by further increasing the rate and completeness of thrombolysis. It appears that this pharmacological approach is capable of converting an acutely unstable coronary lesion into a more predictable stenosis that may be treated utilizing the well-established guidelines of chronic angina.

ACKNOWLEDGMENTS

We acknowledge the close association with Jennifer Johns, M.B., B.S., Tsunehiro Yasuda, M.D., Harry Garabedian, S.M., and Désiré Collen, M.D., Ph.D., all of whom were critical for the development of these ideas. We are grateful to Missy Stanton for preparation of the manuscript.

REFERENCES

1. Collen D, Topol EJ, Tiefenbrunn AJ, Gold HK, Weisfeldt ML, Sobel BE, Leinbach RC, Brinker JA, Ludbrook PA, Yasuda T, Bulkley BH, Robison AK, Hutter AM, Bell WR, Spadaro JJ, Khaw BA, Grossbard EB: Coronary thrombolysis with recombinant human tissue-type plasminogen activator: a prospective, randomized, placebo-controlled trial. Circulation 70:1012, 1984.

2. The TIMI Study Group: The thrombolysis in myocardial infarction (TIMI) trial: phase I findings. N Engl J Med 312:832, 1985.

3. Verstraete M, Bernard R, Bory M, Brower RW, Collen D, DeBono DP, Erbel R, Huhmann W, Lennane RJ, Lubsen J, Mathey D, Meyer J, Michels HR, Rutsch W, Schartl M, Schmidt W, Uebis R, von Essen R: Randomized trial of intravenous recombinant tissue-type plasminogen activator versus intravenous streptokinase in acute myocardial infarction. Lancet 1:842, 1985.

4. Chesebro JH, Smith HC, Holmes DR, Bove AA, Bresnahan DR, Gresnahan JF, Gibbons RJ, Miller PA, Mock, Reeder GS, Vlietstra RE, Brown BC: Reocclusion and clot lysis between 90 minutes, 1 day, and 10 days after thrombolytic therapy for myocardial infarction. Circulation 72:II-55, 1985.

5. Gold HK, Leinbach RC, Garabedian HD, Yasuda T, Johns JA, Grossbard EB, Palacios I, Collen D: Acute coronary reocclusion after thrombolysis with recombinant human tissue-type plasminogen activator: prevention by a maintenance infusion. Circulation 73(2):347, 1986.

6. Garabedian HD, Gold HK, Leinbach RC, Johns JA, Yasuda T, Kanuke M, Collen D: Comparative properties of two clinical preparations of recombinant human tissue-type plasminogen activator in patients with acute myocardial infarction. Submitted for publication.

7. Brown BG, Bolsom EL, Fremir M, Dodge HT: Quantitative coronary arteriography: Estimation of dimensions, hemodynamic resistance, and atheroma mass of coronary artery lesions using the arteriogram and digital computation. Circulation 55:329, 1977.

8. Meyer J, Merx W, Schmitz H, et al: Percutaneous transluminal coronary angioplasty immediately after intracoronary streptolysis of transmural myocardial infarction. Circulation 66:905, 1983.

9. Hartzler GO, Rutherford BD, McConahay DR, Johnson WL, McCallister BD, Gura GM, Conn RC, Crockette JE: Percutaneous transluminal coronary angioplasty with and without thrombolytic therapy for treatment of acute myocardial infarction. Am Heart J 106:965, 1983.

10. Merz W, Dorr R, Rentrop P, Blanke H, Karsch KR, Mathey DG, Kremer P, Rutsch W, Schmutzler H: Evaluation of the effectiveness of intracoronary streptokinase infusion in acute myocardial infarction: postprocedure management and hospital course in 204 patients. Am Heart J 102:1181, 1981.

11. Ganz W, Geft I, Shah PK, Lew AS, Rodriguez L, Weiss T, Maddahi J, Berman DS, Cheruzi Y, Swan HJC: Intravenous streptokinase in evolving acute myocardial infarction. Am J Cardiol 53:1209, 1984.

12. Fox KAA, Robison AK, Knabb RM, Rosamond TL, Sobel BE, Bergmann SR: Prevention of coronary thrombosis with subthrombolytic doses of tissue-type plasminogen activator. Circulation 71:1346, 1985.
13. Laffel GL, Braunwald E: Thrombolytic therapy: a new strategy for the treatment of acute myocardial infarction (first of two parts). N Engl J Med 311(11):710, 1984.
14. Rovelli F, Vita CD, Feruglio GA, Lotto A, Selvini A, Tognoni G: Effectiveness of intravenous thrombolytic treatment in acute myocardial infarction. GISSI Study Group. Lancet 1:397, 1986.

VENOUS THROMBOEMBOLISM AND PERIPHERAL VASCULAR OCCLUSION

8

Thrombolytic Therapy in Venous Thromboembolism

Alexander G. G. Turpie
McMaster University
and Hamilton General Hospital
Hamilton, Ontario, Canada

I. INTRODUCTION

Venous thrombosis and pulmonary embolism usually occur as common and serious complications of medical and surgical patients in hospitals but may affect otherwise healthy ambulant individuals. In the majority of patients, venous thrombosis in the lower limbs begins in the veins of the calf and may remain localized, producing few if any symptoms and no significant long-term consequences. In approximately half of these patients, pulmonary emboli will occur, but these are usually small and well tolerated. In 20% of patients with calf vein thrombosis, the thrombi will extend into the popliteal and more proximal veins, and in 40% of these patients, pulmonary emboli will develop that may be fatal (1). Calf vein thrombi often resolve, but once there has been extension into the more proximal vessels, complete resolution is less likely. Nearly two-thirds of these patients will have residual thrombosis and loss of venous valve function, which produces altered venous return and, in some patients, symptoms and signs of the postphlebitic syndrome, including leg swelling, pigmentation, and ulceration (2).

In patients with symptomatic pulmonary embolism, fatal pulmonary embolism is likely to occur in approximately 20% of untreated patients. In almost all of these patients, death is from recurrent embolism, and at autopsy there is evidence of prior emboli in more than 75% of patients (3). In high-risk hospitalized patients, fatal pulmonary embolism remains the most common preventable cause of death in hospitals and is responsible for approximately 150,000–200,000 deaths per year in the United States (4).

Since progression and embolization of venous thrombi may occur rapidly and unpredictably, it is imperative that all patients in whom the presence of deep vein thrombosis or pulmonary embolism has been confirmed should receive prompt antithrombotic therapy. Heparin is the treatment of choice in most patients with venous thromboembolic disease. With treatment, the outlook for survival and recovery is excellent. Progression or embolization occurs in less than 5% of patients with deep vein thrombosis treated with heparin. In patients with pulmonary embolism treated with heparin, the recurrence rate is less than 5% with a very low mortality, and even in patients with massive embolization or shock, mortality is less than 20% (5,6). However, it should be emphasized that safe, effective methods of prophylaxis against deep vein thrombosis and pulmonary embolism are now available and should be used in all high-risk patients to prevent death and morbidity from venous thromboembolism. Prophylaxis is much more cost-effective than treating the established disease (7).

II. THROMBOLYTIC THERAPY

Anticoagulant therapy is effective in most patients with venous thromboembolic disease, but on theoretical grounds it is not ideal because it does not produce significant thrombolysis. Therefore, although it is effective in reducing the important immediate complications of venous thromboembolism, it may be relatively ineffective in preventing some of the late sequelae.

Thrombolytic therapy has a number of potential advantages over anticoagulant therapy. In the deep venous system of the legs, these advantages include lysis of thrombi with restoration of the circulation to normal, reduction or prevention of venous valve damage, and the potential for preventing the postphlebitic syndrome. In the pulmonary arterial tree, the advantages include rapid reduction of hemodynamic disturbances and prevention or reduction in damage of the pulmonary vascular bed, which may reduce the likelihood of chronic thromboembolic pulmonary hypertension. In addition, there is evidence from clinical studies that thrombolytic therapy may be more effective than anticoagulants in patients with acute massive venous thrombosis or massive pulmonary embolism. For these reasons, thrombolytic therapy is being increasingly used in the initial management of patients with deep vein thrombosis and pulmonary embolism.

There are two major classes of thrombolytic drugs: the plasminogen activators, which convert plasminogen to plasmin, and the proteolytic enzymes such as plasmin, which hydrolyses fibrin directly. Of these, only the plasminogen activators have undergone extensive clinical testing (8–10).

Both streptokinase and urokinase have been used extensively in humans in the treatment of venous thromboembolic disease. However, because both drugs convert plasminogen to plasmin, either directly or indirectly in the circulation, they may give rise to a systemic lytic state. Plasmin exerts proteolytic activity in plasma, leading to depletion of fibrinogen and plasminogen along with consumption of alpha$_2$-antiplasmin. In addition, the breakdown products of fibrinogen, fibrinogen degradation products (FDPs), accumulate, exerting an anticoagulant action. The profound coagulopathy produced may give rise to excessive bleeding that might be quite persistent (11).

Deep Vein Thrombosis

Thrombolytic therapy with streptokinase has been evaluated in a number of small studies in deep vein thrombosis and it has been shown to produce greater lysis of deep vein thrombi than does heparin. However, whether thrombolytic therapy reduces the frequency of the postphlebitic syndrome in these patients has not been established.

There have been six properly designed randomized trials comparing intravenous streptokinase with heparin in the treatment of deep vein thrombosis using thrombolysis on repeat venography as the major endpoint (12–17). None of the trials was large enough to adequately determine both the efficacy and the safety of streptokinase. However, a pooled analysis (18) demonstrated that thrombolysis was achieved approximately four times more often among patients treated with streptokinase than among patients treated with heparin (p < 0.001). Only three of the trials had sufficient data to allow comparison of bleeding complications, which occurred approximately three times more often in the streptokinase group compared with the heparin group (12,16,17).

There have been few properly designed trials of urokinase in venous thrombosis, but clinical reports indicate similar lysis to streptokinase (10).

There have also been few reports on the long-term effects of thrombolytic therapy in deep vein thrombosis. In a large-scale prospective trial recently reported, the frequency of the postphlebitic syndrome was not lower in patients treated with streptokinase compared with heparin after more than 5 years of followup (19). This, however, has not been the experience reported in other trials (20,21).

Overall, the evidence indicates that thrombolytic therapy has great potential in the management of patients with deep vein thrombosis.

Pulmonary Embolism

Most patients with acute pulmonary embolism can be treated successfully with conventional anticoagulant therapy (3,7). In some patients, however, acute pulmonary embolism compromises cardiorespiratory function, and in these patients thrombolytic therapy may be life-saving.

The results of controlled trials have demonstrated that both streptokinase and urokinase are more effective than heparin in inducing rapid resolution of pulmonary emboli. However, the studies were not large enough to demonstrate any effect on mortality (22). These studies (23,24), involving more than 300 patients with pulmonary embolism, demonstrated that treatment with urokinase for either 12 or 24 hr or with streptokinase for 24 hr was more effective than heparin in promoting early resolution of pulmonary embolism. The results showed that with thrombolytic drugs, there was a greater mean reduction in angiographic size of emboli and a greater reduction in perfusion defect demonstrated by lung scanning compared with heparin treatment. In addition, there was some evidence that thrombolytic therapy produced significant benefit in a number of hemodynamic parameters, including pulmonary artery pressure and total pulmonary vascular resistance (25). In these studies, there were no significant differences between the effectiveness of urokinase given for 12 to 24 hours than streptokinase given for 24 hours (23,24).

Followup observations with serial lung scans up to a year after treatment demonstrated that the improvement with thrombolytic therapy was limited to the first week, and thereafter the difference in the rate of lysis between heparin and thrombolytic therapy disappeared. The clinical significance of this finding is unclear (22).

The indications for thrombolytic therapy in patients with acute pulmonary embolism have not been definitely established. The patients most likely to benefit are those with massive pulmonary embolism or preexisting cardiopulmonary disease in whom even a moderate embolism produces severe hemodynamic effects. In both these groups of patients, the rapid lysis of even a moderate amount of embolic material could be life-saving.

III. THROMBOLYTIC THERAPY PROTOCOL

In the treatment of thromboembolic disease, either urokinase or streptokinase may be used, and, although streptokinase is reported to produce a greater frequency of pyrogenic and allergic reactions, there is no convincing evidence that either drug is superior over the other. However, streptokinase is more readily available and is less expensive.

Before thrombolytic therapy is commenced in the treatment of deep vein thrombosis, the diagnosis should be established by objective means such as impedance plethysmography or ascending venography (26). For pulmonary embolism, the diagnosis should be confirmed by pulmonary angiography, but the angiography catheter should be inserted into an arm vein where hemostasis is easier to achieve than it is in the femoral vein (27).

Prior to the commencement of thrombolytic therapy, a baseline prothrombin time, partial thromboplastin time, thrombin clotting time, and platelet count should be obtained, as well as a baseline hemoglobin and hematocrit determination. To minimize the risk of bleeding, invasive arterial procedures should be avoided and venipuncture should be kept to an absolute minimum. If arterial blood samples are required, blood should be taken from the radial artery and local compression maintained for at least 20 min. The effect of thrombolytic therapy may be monitored by tests such as the thrombin clotting time or euglobulin lysis time to establish the presence of a systemic thrombolytic state, but there is no evidence that these tests can predict clinical efficacy or be used to reduce the risk of bleeding (28,29).

Streptokinase should be given in a loading dose of 250,000 U given over 30 min followed by intravenous infusion of 100,000–200,000 U per hour. Monitoring of streptokinase therapy should be performed by carrying out a thrombin clotting time approximately 2 hr after the onset of the loading dose, and the dose of the infusion adjusted accordingly. Once the thrombolytic treatment is established, the thrombin clotting time should be repeated at 4-hr intervals. If the thrombin clotting time remains two to five times the control value, no change in dose is required. Tests of fibrinolytic activity, such as the euglobulin lysis time, may be performed as available but are not necessary. Urokinase should be given in a loading dose of 4400 U/kg over 30 min with a maintenance dose of 4400 U/kg/hr.

The duration of thrombolytic therapy depends on whether it is being used in the management of deep vein thrombosis or pulmonary embolism. In deep vein thrombosis, the period of treatment is usually a minimum of 48 hr, which may be extended to 72 hr. In pulmonary embolism, treatment for 12 to 24 hr is usually all that is required.

After the thrombolytic therapy is discontinued, it should be followed by full-dose therapeutic intravenous heparin followed by secondary prophylaxis with oral anticoagulant therapy (30).

The contraindications to thrombolytic therapy in venous thromboembolic disease include active internal bleeding, recent cerebrovascular accident or other intracranial disease, recent surgery, recent trauma, and severe arterial hypertension. Other relative contraindications include recent minor trauma, including cardiopulmonary resuscitation, bacterial endocarditis, severe hepatorenal disease, and pregnancy. In addition, elderly patients and patients with diabetic haemorrhagic retinopathy should not be given thrombolytic therapy.

IV. COMPLICATIONS OF THROMBOLYTIC THERAPY

The major complication of thrombolytic therapy with streptokinase or urokinase is hemorrhage. Thrombolytic therapy produces lysis of fibrin in hemostatic plugs and wounds and therefore bleeding occurs more frequently than with heparin. The published data suggests that the risk of major hemorrhage with streptokinase is approximately twice that associated with heparin therapy and occurs in 30% or more of patients treated with streptokinase infusions for more than 12 hr. The risk of hemorrhage increases with the length of the infusion and occurs most often in sites of previous surgery or trauma or from sites of vascular invasions, such as needle puncture wounds and cutdown sites for catheterization. In about one-third of patients, bleeding commences during the thrombolytic therapy; in the remaining patients, it is first noted after completion of thrombolytic therapy and during anticoagulant therapy. Bleeding may also occur in the genitourinary or gastrointestinal tracts, and occasionally cerebral bleeding occurs. Bleeding complications can be reduced by carefully selecting patients and not treating those with contraindications.

V. HUMAN TISSUE-TYPE PLASMINOGEN ACTIVATOR

Recently, a new plasminogen activator, extrinsic or tissue-type plasminogen activator (t-PA), which preferentially activates plasminogen in the presence of fibrin, has been isolated from human tissues. The activation process of t-PA is localized to the site of the thrombus, which decreases the degree of generation of a systemic lytic state and thus decreases the accompanying risk of abnormal bleeding. Kinetic analyses suggest that plasminogen activation in the presence of fibrin occurs after binding of plasminogen and tissue-type plasminogen activator to the clot surface. This complex results in an increased concentration of plasmin at the fibrin clot surface. Tissue-type plasminogen activator has been shown in in vitro studies and in vivo studies in animals to produce lysis of venous thrombi with negligible fibrinogen breakdown. Tissue plasminogen activator has now been produced by recombinant DNA technology (rt-PA) with biological properties that are identical to those of naturally occurring t-PA (31).

VI. EXPERIMENTAL STUDIES IN VENOUS THROMBOSIS WITH t-PA

The thrombolytic potential of tissue-type plasminogen activator has been evaluated in several animal models of deep vein thrombosis and pulmonary embolism. In experimental venous thrombosis models in rabbits (32) and dogs (33), rt-PA has been shown to be more effective than streptokinase or urokinase in inducing thrombolysis but—in contrast to streptokinase and urokinase—without producing plasma proteolysis. As experience has accumulated, it has become evident that the fibrin selectivity of rt-PA is relative and is influenced by the dose and duration of the rt-PA infusion. A number of studies in experimental venous thrombosis in animals with rt-PA have been carried out to determine whether dosage regimens of rt-PA can be developed to induce thrombolysis without producing a systemic fibrinogenolytic state with the aim of reducing the risk of excessive hemorrhage (34,35).

In a study of experimental venous thrombosis in rabbits (32), rt-PA in a dose of 7500 U/kg/hr infused over 4 hr produced thrombolysis without inducing systemic fibrinogenolysis and without producing excessive bleeding. At higher doses of rt-PA (15,000 U/kg over 4 hr) there was enhanced thrombolysis, but this was associated with fibrinogenolysis and excessive bleeding. In this study, which compared the thrombolytic and hemorrhagic effects of rt-PA with streptokinase, at thrombolytic doses streptokinase always induced excessive bleeding, while rt-PA did not induce bleeding at the lower dose used, which produced more thrombolysis than streptokinase did. In addition, in contrast to the bleeding induced by streptokinase, which occurred soon after the commencement of the infusion, the bleeding with high-dose rt-PA was delayed for up to 2 hr after starting the rt-PA infusion. Further studies were carried out in experimental venous thrombosis in rabbits to determine the optimum dosage regimen (34,35), on the basis that improved thrombolysis might be maintained by infusing a high-dose of rt-PA over a short period of time. These studies were based on the observation that the thrombolytic effect of rt-PA persisted beyond its time of clearance from the circulation (34) and wound bleeding induced by a high dose of infused rt-PA was delayed for at least 2 hr after starting the infusion (32). The experiments were performed by infusing 30,000 U/kg of rt-PA or saline into rabbits over times ranging from 15 to 240 min, using a jugular vein thrombosis model. The thrombolytic effect of the different dosage regimens of rt-PA was assessed 4 hr after starting the infusion and measured every 15 min for 4 hr. The effect of the different rt-PA dosage regimens on alpha$_2$-antiplasmin, fibrinogen, and the thrombin clotting time were evaluated every 15 min. Compared with saline placebo, 30,000 kg of rt-PA infused over 4 hr, 1 hr, 30 min, and 15 min produced 36, 87, 88, and 96% thrombolysis, respectively. Infusion of t-PA over 1 hr and 4 hr induced a significant increase in blood loss while the 30- and 15-min infusions did not produce more bleeding than did the saline control infusion. The alpha$_2$-antiplasmin levels were significantly reduced with the 1- and 4-hr infusions but were not reduced with the 15- and 30-min infusions. These findings indicate that a rapid infusion regimen results in improved thrombolysis with minimal fibrinogenolysis and without excessive bleeding. In contrast to these findings, a study in rabbits using 20-hr aged thrombi reported that infusion of rt-PA at the same dosage (48,000 U/kg over different periods of time, 240, 90, and 30 min) produced similar degrees of thrombolysis, but no information was provided on bleeding induced by different dosage regimens (36).

In a study of experimental pulmonary embolism in rabbits (37), rt-PA has been shown to be highly effective in producing thrombolysis at lower doses than those of urokinase, without extensive systemic plasminogen activation. Thus, there is evidence for experimental clinical models that rt-PA is highly effective in producing thrombolysis without causing a systemic lytic state, thus reducing the risk of hemorrhage.

VII. t-PA IN HUMAN VENOUS THROMBOEMBOLIC DISEASE

Initial case reports on the use of rt-PA in patients with acute proximal vein thrombosis demonstrated marked thrombolysis with minimal fibrinogenolysis (38).

We have completed two pilot studies evaluating the clinical usefulness of rt-PA in deep vein thrombosis in humans compared with that of heparin alone (39). The specific objectives of the first study were to assess whether a regimen of a 4-hr infusion of recombinant t-PA in doses of 0.5 mg/kg plus standard heparin was more effective than heparin alone in promoting resolution of venographically confirmed proximal deep vein thrombosis when evaluated by repeat venography within 72 hr, to assess whether a second infusion of t-PA in a dose of 0.5 mg/kg over 1 hr was more effective than heparin alone in promoting resolution of proximal deep venous thrombosis evaluated by serial impedance plethysmography, to document the frequency of hemorrhage with combined rt-PA and heparin therapy compared with heparin alone, and to correlate the changes of tests of fibrinolysis to the rates of thrombolysis or bleeding induced by rt-PA.

Twenty-four patients were studied; 12 received rt-PA and 12 received placebo. There was no difference linked to age, sex, or whether the patients had symptomatic or postoperative deep vein thrombosis. Of the 12 patients who received rt-PA, five patients obtained greater than 50% lysis of the thrombi, four patients obtained significant but less than 50% lysis, and three patients showed no evidence of lysis. Figure 1 shows the extent of thrombolysis obtained after a 4-hr infusion of rt-PA in one patient. In contrast, only two patients in the heparin-alone group obtained less than 50% lysis, and 10 patients showed no lysis. It was not possible to evaluate the degree of lysis adequately after the second infusion using impedance plethysmography, although in some patients the test returned to normal. Two patients in the rt-PA group had overt hemorrhage, one had marked bruising, and one patient developed hemarthrosis 10 days after total hip replacement; two patients had a fall in hemoglobin of greater than 20 G/L but without overt bleeding. In the heparin-only group, one patient had a spontaneous hemarthrosis of the shoulder, and one had a fall in hemoglobin of greater than 20 G/L without overt bleeding. The rt-PA infusion produced a fall in circulating fibrinogen concentration to approximately 50% of the preinfusion value, a fall in plasma plasminogen to 60% of the preinfusion value, and a fall in alpha$_2$-antiplasmin to almost undetectable levels. There was a threefold increase in the concentration of serum fibrinogen degradation products. The changes in parameters of fibrinolysis for the 4-hr infusions are shown in Figure 2; identical changes were seen after the 1-hr infusion. Thus, there was a moderate degree of plasmin-induced proteolysis with both the 4- and 1-hr infusions, and a significant number of patients had hemorrhagic complications.

A possible explanation in the decreased concentrations of the various components of fibrinolytic enzyme system is in vitro proteolysis. However, there are two lines of evidence that support the proposition that the results represent an in vivo effect of rt-PA infusion. The observed decrease in the concentration of circulating components of the fibrinolytic enzyme persists, or is even lower, in samples taken 2 hr after the t-PA infusion has been discontinued. Since the half-life of rt-PA is 8 to 9 min in humans, it is difficult to

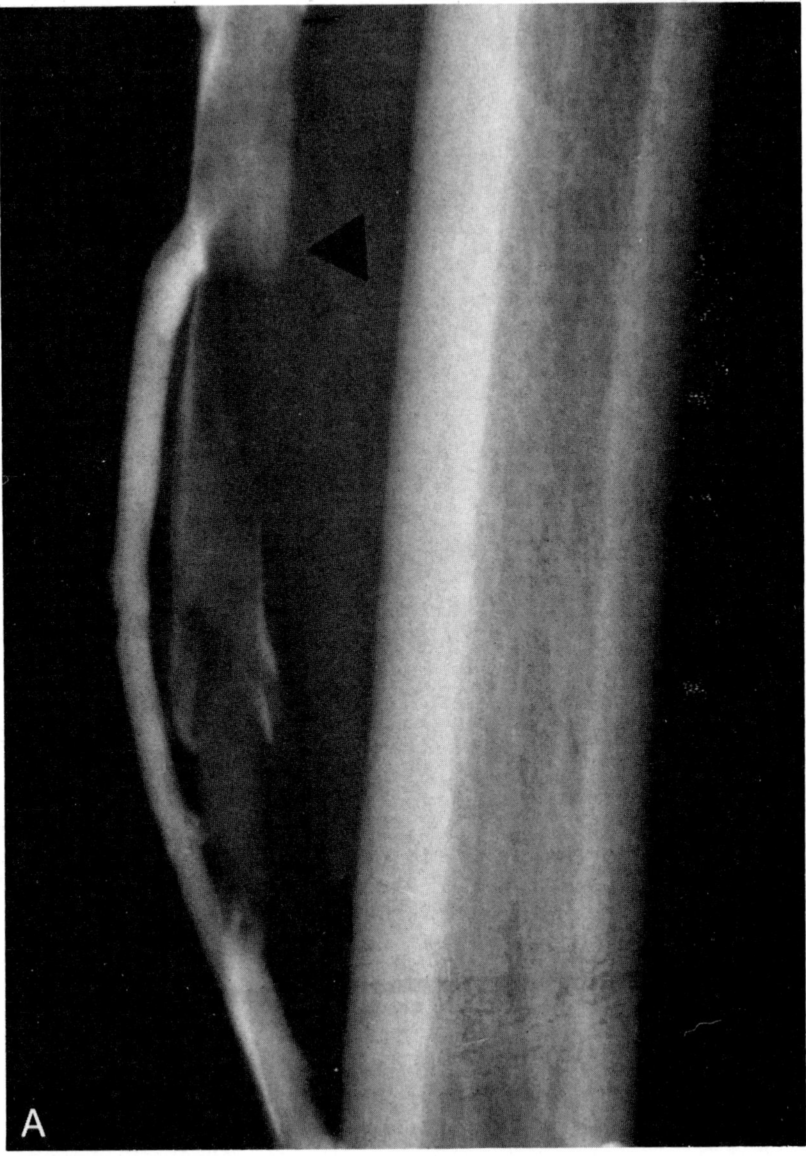

Figure 1   Venography in a patient treated with a 4-hr infusion of rt-PA in a dose of 0.5 mg/kg showing (A) extensive common femoral vein thrombosis before treatment and (B) almost complete thrombolysis after treatment.

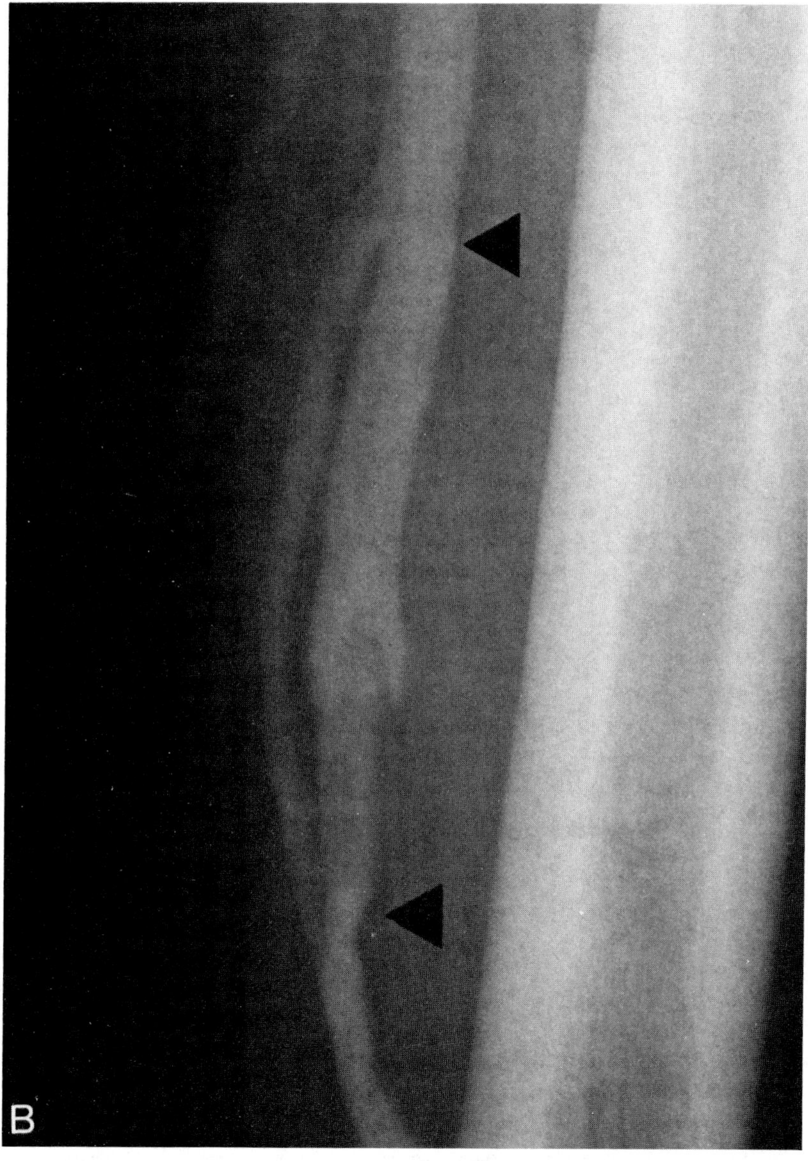

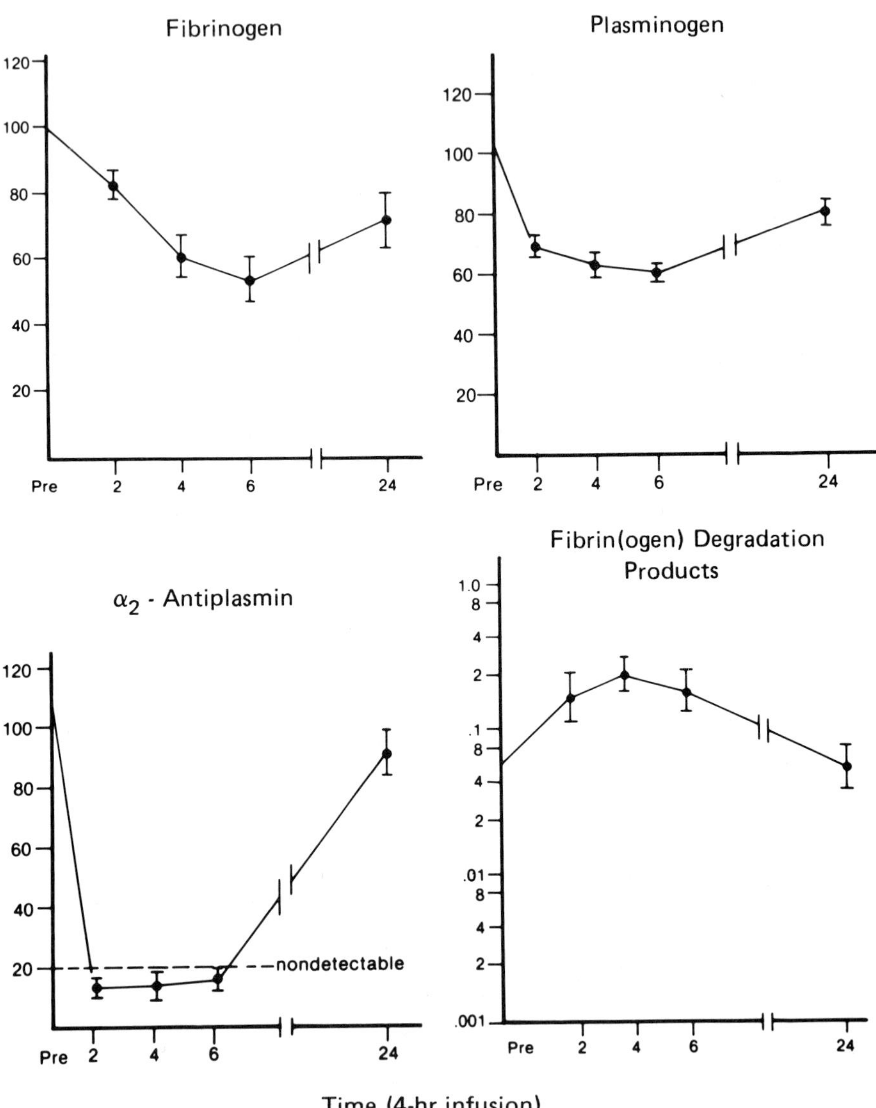

Figure 2   Parameters of fibrinolysis after a 4-hr infusion of 0.5 mg/kg rt-PA. Data from 10 patients with proximal vein thrombosis shown as mean percentage of preinfusion value for fibrinogen, plasminogen, α_2-antiplasmin, and G/L for fibrinogen degradation products.

attribute the persistently low levels detected 2 hr after infusion to an in vitro effect. Secondly, alpha$_2$-antiplasmin is the parameter least likely to be affected by in vitro proteolysis, yet these results demonstrate that there was a more dramatic and persistent reduction of alpha$_2$-antiplasmin to nondetectable levels. The results are, therefore, consistent with the hypothesis that significant amounts of plasmin were generated initially to deplete alpha$_2$-antiplasmin and subsequently to cause plasmin-induced proteolysis. The results of this study indicate that t-PA combined with heparin treatment produced significantly more lysis in proximal deep vein thrombosis than did heparin alone, but the dosage regimen used produced a moderate degree of plasmin-induced proteolysis and was associated with a significant number of hemorrhagic complications.

We therefore compared a second dosage regimen of rt-PA with heparin in which patients treated with intravenous heparin received two 8-hr infusions of rt-PA in a dose of 0.5 mg/kg given 24 hr apart. Twenty patients were studied, ten in the t-PA-plus-heparin group and ten in the heparin-placebo group. Similar results to those of the first study were obtained in terms of thrombolytic and hemorrhagic effects. Six of the ten patients treated with rt-PA showed greater than 50% lysis, one showed less than 50%, and three showed no evidence of lysis. No patients in the heparin group showed evidence of thrombolysis. Three of the ten patients in the rt-PA-treated group had spontaneous hemorrhages, compared with none in the heparin group. In marked contrast to the first study, there was minimal reduction in the indices of thrombolysis. These results are shown in Table 1. This raises the possibility that factors other than fibrinogenolysis may be responsible for rt-PA-associated hemorrhage.

Tissue plasminogen activator has been shown in case reports and small descriptive studies (40,41) to produce dramatic lysis of acute pulmonary

Table 1   Indices of Lytic Activity After 8-hr Infusion of 0.5 mg/kg rT-PA in Six Patients with DVT (Mean ± SD)

	rT-PA		Placebo	
	Preinfusion	2-hr postinfusion	Preinfusion	2-hr postinfusion
Fibrinogen G/L	4.11 ± 1.10	3.60 ± 1.30	3.60 ± 1.00	3.70 ± 1.50
Alpha$_2$-antiplasmin (%)	1.13 ± 0.12	0.42 ± 0.30	1.12 ± 0.34	1.10 ± 0.22
FDP G/L	0.04 ± 0.04	0.27 ± 0.29	0.03 ± 0.02	0.03 ± 0.04

embolism without significant fibrinogenolysis or bleeding. Major studies of
t-PA in acute pulmonary embolism are in progress.

VIII. CONCLUSION

The two dosage regimens of rt-PA that have been evaluated in deep vein
thrombosis produced highly significant thrombolysis, but they are not optimal
because they produce excessive bleeding. It is clear that the therapeutic range
for rt-PA in humans for the treatment of deep vein thrombosis remains to be
determined. The ideal dosage regimen for rt-PA should achieve effective
thrombolysis quickly with minimal fibrinogenolysis to minimize bleeding. It
should be possible to optimize the dosage regimen by carrying out carefully
controlled clinical trials in patients with human thromboembolic disease. This
work was supported by Medical Research Grant of Canada MA-9290.

REFERENCES

1. Kakkar VV, Flank C, Howe CT, et al: Natural history of postoperative deep vein
    thrombosis. Lancet 2:230–233, 1969.
2. Negus D: The post-thrombotic syndrome. Ann R Coll Surg Engl 47:92–105,
    1970.
3. Morrell MP, Dunhill MS: The postmortem incidence of pulmonary embolism in a
    hospital population. Br J Surg 55:347, 1968.
4. Coon WW, Willis PW, Keller JB: Thromboembolism and other venous disease
    in the Tecumseh Community Health Study. Circulation 48:839–846, 1973.
5. Barritt DW, Jordan SC: Anticoagulant drugs in the treatment of pulmonary
    embolism: A controlled clinical trial. Lancet 1:1309–1312, 1960.
6. Kanis JA: Heparin in the treatment of pulmonary thromboembolism. Thrombos
    Diathes Haemorrh 32:519–527, 1974.
7. Salzman EW, Hirsh J: Prevention of venous thromboembolism. In *Hemostasis
    and Thrombosis*: *Basic Principles and Clinical Practice*, Colman RW, Hirsh J,
    Marder VJ, Salzman EW, Eds., Lippincott, Philadelphia, 1982. pp. 986–999.
8. Fratantoni JC, Ness P, Simon TL: Thrombolytic therapy. Current status. N Engl
    J Med 293:1073, 1975.
9. Kakkar VV, Scully MF: Thrombolytic therapy. Br Med Bull 34:191, 1978.
10. Thrombolytic therapy in thrombosis: A National Institutes of Health Consensus
    Development Conference. Ann Intern Med 93:141–144, 1980.
11. Verstraete M: Biochemical and clinical aspects of thrombolysis. Semin Hematol
    15:35, 1978.
12. Robertson BR, Nilsson IM, Nylander G: Value of streptokinase and heparin in
    treatment of acute deep venous thrombosis: a coded investigation. Acta Chir
    Scand 134:203–208, 1968.
13. Kakkar VV, Flanc C, Howe CT, O'Shea M, Flute PT: Treatment of deep vein

thrombosis: a trial of heparin, streptokinase, and arvin. Br Med J 1:806–810, 1969.

14. Robertson BR, Nilsson IM, Nylander G: Thrombolytic effect of streptokinase as evaluated by phlebography of deep venous thrombi of the leg. Acta Chir Scand 136:173–180, 1970.

15. Tsapogas MJ, Peabody RA, Wu KT, Karmody AM, Devaraj KT, Eckert C: Controlled study of thrombolytic therapy in deep vein thrombosis. Surgry 74: 973–985, 1973.

16. Porter JM, Seaman AJ, Common HH, Rosch J, Eidemiller LR, Calhoun AD: Comparison of heparin and streptokinase in the treatment of venous thrombosis. Am Surg 41:511–519, 1975.

17. Elliott MS, Immelman EJ, Jeffrey P, Benatar SR, Funston MR, Smith JA, Shepstone BJ, Ferguson AD, Jacobs P, Walker W, Louw JH: A comparative randomized trial of heparin versus streptokinase in the treatment of acute proximal venous thrombosis: an interim report of a prospective trial. Br J Surg 66:838–843, 1979.

18. Goldhaber SZ, Buring JE, Lipnick RJ, Hennekens CH: Pooled analyses of randomized trials of streptokinase and heparin in phlebographically documented acute deep venous thrombosis. Am J Med 76:393–397, 1984.

19. Kakkar VV, Paes TRF, Murray WJG: Does thrombolytic therapy prevent the post-phlebitic syndrome? Thrombosis Haemostasis 54(abstr):175, 1985.

20. Common HH, Seaman AJ, Rosch J, Porter JM, Dotter CT: Deep vein thrombosis treated with streptokinase or heparin. Follow-up of a randomized study. Angiology 27:645, 1976.

21. Johansson E, Ericson K, Zetterquist S: Streptokinase treatment of deep venous thrombosis of the lower extremity. Acta Med Scand 199:89, 1976.

22. Genton E: Thrombolytic therapy of pulmonary thromboembolism. Prog Cardiovasc Dis 21:333, 1979.

23. Urokinase-Pulmonary Embolism Trial. Phase I results. JAMA 214:2163, 1970.

24. Urokinase-Streptokinase Embolism Trial. Phase II results. A Coooperative Study. JAMA 299:1606, 1974.

25. Sharma GVRK, Burleson VA, Sasahara AA: Effect of thrombolytic therapy on pulmonary capillary blood volume in patients with pulmonary embolism. N Engl J Med 303:842, 1980.

26. Hull R, Hirsh J: Diagnosis of venous thrombosis. In *Hemostasis and Thrombosis: Basic Principles and Clinical Practice*, Colman RW, Hirsh J, Marder VJ, Salzman EW, Eds., Lippincott, Philadelphia, 1982, pp. 844–856.

27. Hull RD, Hirsh J, Carter CJ, Jay RM, Dodd PE, Ockleford PA, Coates G, Gill GJ, Turpie AGG, et al: Pulmonary angiography, ventilation lung scanning and venography for clinically suspected pulmonary embolism with abnormal perfusion lung scan. Ann Intern Med 98:891–899, 1983.

28. Marder VJ: The use of thrombolytic agents: Choice of patient, drug administration, laboratory monitoring. Ann Intern Med 90:802, 1979.

29. Bell WR, Meek AG: Guidelines for the use of thrombolytic agents. N Engl J Med 301: 1266, 1979.

30. Hull R, Hirsh J, Jay R, Carter CJ, England C, Gent M, Turpie AGG, McLaughlin D, Dodd P, Thomas M, Raskob G, Ockelford P: Different intensities of oral anticoagulant therapy in the treatment of proximal vein thrombosis. N Engl J Med 307:1676–1681, 1982.

31. Pennica D, Holmes WE, Kohr WJ, Harkins RN, Vehar GA, Ward CA, Bennett WF, Yelverton E, Seeburg PH, Heyneker HL, Goeddel DV, Collen D: Cloning and expression of human tissue-type plasminogen activator cDNA in *E. coli.* Nature 301:214–221, 1983.

32. Agnelli G, Buchanan MR, Fernandez F, Boneu B, VanRyn J, Hirsh J, Collen D: A comparison of the thrombolytic and hemorrhagic effects of tissue-type plasminogen activator and streptokinase in rabbits. Circulation 72:178–182, 1985.

33. Korninger C, Matsuo O, Suy R, Stassen JM, Collen D: Thrombolysis with human extrinsic (tissue-type) plasminogen activator. J Clin Invest 69:573–580, 1982.

34. Agnelli G, Buchanan MR, Fernandez F, VanRyn J, Hirsh J: Sustained thrombolysis with DNA-recombinant tissue type plasminogen activator in rabbits. Blood 66:399–401, 1985.

35. Agnelli G, Buchanan MR, Fernandez F, Hirsh J: The thrombolytic and hemorrhagic effects of tissue type plasminogen activator: Influence of dosage regimens in rabbits. Throm Res 40:769–777, 1985.

36. Collen D, Stassen JM, Marafino BJ Jr, Builder S, DeCock F, Ogez J, Tijiri D, Pennica D, Bennett WF, Salwa J, Hoyng CF: Biological properties of human tissue-type plasminogen activator obtained by expression of recombinant DNA in mammalian cells. J Pharmacol Exp Ther 23:146–152, 1984.

37. Matsuo O, Rijken C, Collen D: Thrombolysis by human tissue plasminogen activator and urokinase in rabbits with experimental pulmonary embolus. Nature 291:590–591, 1981.

38. Weimar W, Stibbe J, van Seyen A, Biliau P, DeSomer P, Collen D: Specific lysis of an iliofemoral thrombus by administration of extrinsic (tissue-type) plasminogen activator. Lancet 2:1018–1020, 1981.

39. Turpie AGG, Jay RM, Carter CJ, Hirsh J: A randomized trial of recombinant tissue plasminogen activator for the treatment of proximal deep vein thrombosis. Circulation II-72(abstr 770), 1985.

40. Bounameaux H, Vermylen J, Collen D: Thrombolytic treatment with recombinant tissue-type plasminogen activator in a patient with massive pulmonary embolism. Ann Intern Med 103:64–65, 1985.

41. Goldhaber SZ, Vaughan DE, Markis JE, Selwyn AP, Meyerovitz M, Dawley L, Kim DS, Loscalzo J, Sasahara A, Benotti J, Grossbard EB, Braunwald E: Efficacy and safety of tissue plasminogen activator in the treatment of acute pulmonary embolism. J Am Coll Cardiol 7(abstr):68A, 1986.

9

Tissue Plasminogen Activators in the Treatment of Acute Pulmonary Embolism

Samuel Z. Goldhaber and Eugene Braunwald
Harvard Medical School
and Brigham and Women's Hospital
Boston, Massachusetts

I. INTRODUCTION

Pulmonary embolism (PE) is a common cardiovascular disorder that is often precipitated by deep venous thrombosis (DVT) and that can cause pulmonary hypertension, right ventricular dysfunction, or death. Despite a decrease in the mortality rate from PE in the early and mid 1970s (1), data from the National Center for Health Statistics suggest that during the past decade the case fatality rate for PE as a primary discharge diagnosis has remained approximately 14%, with essentially no further improvement (2).

Standard therapy for PE has employed heparin anticoagulation followed by warfarin, without thrombolytic therapy. The rationale for anticoagulation therapy is to provide prophylaxis against additional thromboembolic events while natural fibrinolytic mechanisms gradually lyse the previously formed pulmonary artery clot. In contrast, the rationale for thrombolytic therapy (followed by anticoagulation) is that thrombolysis actively dissolves clot that has already formed, thereby restoring cardiopulmonary function to normal as quickly as possible. Thrombolysis relieves the obstruction to pulmonary artery blood flow and thus improves right ventricular function, reduces pulmonary artery pressures, and ameliorates pulmonary tissue perfusion. Thrombolytic therapy may also reduce the frequency of chronic pulmonary hypertension as a result of PE.

The hemodynamic response to PE depends upon the size of the embolus, coexistent cardiopulmonary disease, and neurohumoral responses. When acute PE obstructs pulmonary artery blood flow, right ventricular afterload increases. In patients without prior cardiopulmonary disease, right ventricular pressure increases when approximately 25% of the pulmonary blood flow is obstructed. Right ventricular systolic pressure continues to rise as the degree of obstruction increases. During the acute event, the previously unstressed normal right ventricle cannot usually generate a maximum mean pulmonary artery pressure that exceeds 30 mm Hg. As afterload continues to increase, the right ventricle begins to fail and right atrial pressure rises. When forward cardiac output can no longer be sustained, clinical shock ensues.

II. THROMBOLYTIC THERAPY VS. ANTICOAGULATION

For patients with major PE who are treated with anticoagulation therapy alone, complete resolution of pulmonary artery clot may fail to occur in 75% of patients after 1–4 weeks (3) and in 50% after 4 months (4) of followup. Efforts to evaluate thrombolytic therapy versus anticoagulation must rely on five published comparisons (5–9), comprising a total of only 210 randomized patients (5,8,9). All studies demonstrated more rapid anatomical or physiological improvement among patients treated with thrombolytic agents. However, no study detected significant differences in mortality, possibly due to the low rate of mortality among control subjects (10) and the small sample size (11), i.e., a Type II error.

The relatively large Phase I portion of the Urokinase Pulmonary Embolism Trial (UPET) sponsored by the National Heart, Lung, and Blood Institute warrants special comment. UPET was a randomized comparison of heparin and urokinase (UK) in 160 patients with angiographically demonstrated PE. Patients received followup hemodynamic, angiographic, and nuclear studies. One day after initiation of therapy, the UK-treated patients exhibited significantly greater hemodynamic and anatomical improvement than did the heparin-treated patients. However, within 5 to 7 days of treatment, no difference between the two groups could be demonstrated on lung scans. During the 2 weeks following therapy, recurrent PE occurred less often among UK-treated patients, 17% versus 23%, but this difference did not achieve statistical significance (12). However, patients treated with UK or streptokinase (SK) have been shown to have improved pulmonary capillary blood volume and pulmonary diffusion capacity compared with patients who received standard heparin anticoagulation (13). Lytic therapy may also remove or reduce the source of the embolus in the venous system, in addition to lysing emboli in the pulmonary artery. Therefore, thrombolytic therapy might hypothetically enable one to shorten safely the duration of conventional heparin and warfarin therapy after administering the lytic agent. UK-treated patients in Phase I of UPET had a 27% frequency of severe bleeding, defined as a fall in hematocrit greater than 10% (e.g., 45% to 34% or less) and/or requiring a blood transfusion of more than two units (5). UK-treated patients in Phase II of UPET had a 12% rate of severe bleeding (14). The excessive bleeding in these patients may be due to the activation by UK and SK of both circulating and fibrin-bound plasminogen, thereby causing systemic fibrinogen depletion.

Although UK and SK were approved for treatment of PE in 1977, their use did not become as widespread as initially predicted. In 1980, an NIH Consensus Development Conference suggested that thrombolytic agents were not being used often enough for patients with PE who: 1) had obstruction of blood flow to a lobe or multiple pulmonary segments or 2) were hemodynamically compromised, regardless of the anatomical size of the PE (15). Nevertheless, use of thrombolytic therapy for PE has continued to languish, whereas administration of lytic therapy for myocardial infarction has been demonstrated to reduce mortality (16,17) and is being used with increasing frequency.

The development of tissue-type plasminogen activator produced by recombinant techniques (rt-PA), a second-generation thrombolytic agent with relative fibrin specificity, has led to reexamiantion of the role of lytic therapy in venous thromboembolism (18).

III. t-PA IN EXPERIMENTAL VENOUS THROMBOEMBOLISM

The thrombolytic effect of melanoma-derived t-PA was compared with that of UK in a canine venous thrombosis model, using the superficial femoral vein (19). Acute venous thrombosis in a 4-cm vein segment was induced by formation of an I-125-fibrinogen-labeled blood clot. Thrombolytic therapy was administered through a peripheral vein. In separate experiments, t-PA and UK were administered as a bolus (10% of the total dose) followed by a continuous intravenous infusion over 4 hr. The degree of thrombolysis was determined by measuring the quantity of radioactivity in the vein segment after thrombolytic therapy, compared with the amount of radioactivity originally incorporated in the clot. The percent lysis of venous clot was 50% greater with 1 mg of double-chain t-PA compared with 1,000,000 IU of UK. Yet, dogs that received t-PA had essentially no fibrinogen depletion. In contrast, dogs that received 1,000,000 IU of UK had complete defibrinogenation and profuse bleeding from their surgical wounds.

UK and melanoma-derived t-PA were also compared in a venous thrombosis model in rabbits (20) that was similar to the dog model and utilized a 4-cm segment of rabbit jugular vein. The total dose of each agent was administered over 4 hr with 10% of the dose given as an initial bolus, followed by a continuous intravenous infusion. When 1 mg of systemically administered single- or double-chain t-PA was compared with 500,000 IU of systemically administered UK, the percent thrombolysis of fresh clot was more than 50% greater among t-PA-treated rabbits. Rabbits that received t-PA had essentially no fibrinogen depletion, whereas rabbits that received 500,000 IU of UK had a 35% reduction of fibrinogen. When 0.2 mg of locally infused t-PA was compared with 100,000 IU of locally infused UK, the percent lysis of 1- and 3-day old clot was twice as great among t-PA-treated rabbits.

Using a similar rabbit model of jugular venous thrombosis, melanoma-derived t-PA was compared with SK for thrombolytic effect and quantitation of hemorrhage (21). Rabbits received systemic intravenous t-PA or SK with 10% of the total dose of the agent administered as a bolus and the remaining 90% infused continuously over the subsequent 4 hr. t-PA, 0.075 and 0.15 mg/kg/hr, produced 35% and 85% lysis, respectively, whereas SK, 8,000 and 16,000 U/kg/hr, produced 28% and 57% thrombolysis, respectively. The higher dose of SK caused profuse bleeding from all wound sites. The lower dose of SK produced approximately 7 times more bleeding than the higher dose of t-PA, even though the percentage decrease of α_2-antiplasmin activity (a marker for a systemic plasmin-mediated proteolytic state) was similar for these two lytic regimens. Bleeding with the lower dose of SK occurred within 15 min of initiating the infusion, compared with the higher dose of t-PA that caused no excess in bleeding until 2 hr after the beginning of the infusion. The lower dose of t-PA caused no excess in bleeding.

Thus, in these experimental models of venous thrombosis, t-PA caused more fibrin-specific thrombolysis and less hemorrhage than did either UK or SK. Melanoma-derived t-PA has also been compared with UK in a rabbit model of PE (22). In this model, an I-125-fibrinogen-labeled thrombus 1.5 cm in length was prepared in a polyethylene tube. The thrombus was then injected through the rabbit jugular vein. The degree of thrombolysis was calculated as the difference in radioactivity between the injected thrombus and the thrombus recovered from postmortem dissection of the pulmonary artery.

As in the previous experiments, 10% of the total dose of the lytic agent was injected into a systemic vein as an initial bolus and the remaining 90% was given as a continuous intravenous infusion. Administration of 1,000,000 IU of UK over 6 hr caused thrombolysis of 12% of the clot, compared with 0.35 mg of t-PA over 6 hr, which caused lysis of 16%, and with 0.7 mg of t-PA over 12 hr, which caused lysis of 23%. The fibrinogen level decreased 30% among the UK-treated rabbits but remained unchanged among the rabbits that received t-PA. These experiments in dogs and rabbits have served as the basis for clinical use of t-PA in patients with venous thromboembolism.

IV. t-PA IN PATIENTS WITH VENOUS THROMBOSIS

The first clinical report of venous thrombosis treated with (melanoma-derived) t-PA was published in 1981 (23). A 30-year-old woman had received a cadaveric renal allograft 2 years previously. Six weeks prior to treatment with t-PA, she presented with extensive unilateral leg edema and a creatinine clearance reduced to 35 ml/min. Venography $2\frac{1}{2}$ weeks later demonstrated thrombosis of the renal and iliofemoral veins. During the subsequent $3\frac{1}{2}$ weeks, she was treated with oral anticoagulation. Because her leg edema and renal function did not improve, she was treated with 7.5 mg of t-PA as a continuous peripheral infusion over 24 hr. Fibrinogen levels remained stable throughout the infusion. On the day following t-PA therapy, a repeat venogram showed recanalization of the iliofemoral vein and disappearance of the renal vein thrombosis compared with the venogram $3\frac{1}{2}$ weeks prior to t-PA treatment. Within the next 2 days the patient's leg edema resolved.

Subsequently, a 73-year-old man was treated with melanoma-derived t-PA for inferior vena caval, right renal vein, and iliofemoral thromboses (23). He received 5 mg of t-PA over 24 hr, with resolution of the clots and improvement in serum creatinine from 4.1 to 2.0 mg/dl. As with the first patient, the fibrinogen level remained stable and there was no evidence of a systemic lytic state.

A randomized, placebo-controlled trial of therapy for angiographically documented DVT included 12 patients assigned to treatment with rt-PA and 12 who received placebo (24). The rt-PA-treated patients received 0.5 mg/kg of rt-PA as a 4-hr continuous intravenous infusion. During and after the 4-hr infusion, both the rt-PA- and the placebo-treated groups received heparin. Venography was repeated 48 to 72 hr after rt-PA or placebo treatment. Overall, five of the 12 rt-PA-treated patients had 50–90% clot lysis, as judged by repeated venography; four had less than 50% lysis; and three had no detectable lysis. Two of the 12 patients who received placebo (followed by heparin) had <50% clot lysis and 10 had no lysis. Among those who received rt-PA, fibrinogen levels decreased by an average of 57% and one patient had a major bleeding complication (hemarthrosis of the hip). In a subsequent randomized trial of 20 DVT patients, extending the duration of the infusion to 8 hr and administering a second 8-hr rt-PA infusion of 0.5 mg/kg prior to repeat venography did not appear to improve the efficacy or safety of rt-PA.

V. rt-PA IN PATIENTS WITH PE

The use of rt-PA in acute PE was first reported in a 63-year-old man with massive PE (documented angiographically) who had undergone renal transplantation 5 weeks before treatment (25). Through a catheter inserted into the right ventricle, 30 mg (0.5 mg/kg) of rt-PA was infused over 90 min. Angiography was repeated 24 hr after rt-PA and demonstrated marked recanalization. Immediately after treatment, the patient felt dramatic subjective improvement, and arterial PO_2 on room air increased from 37 mm Hg before therapy to 66 mm Hg. There were no bleeding complications and the fibrinogen levels remained unchanged.

In our evaluation of the efficacy of rt-PA in acute PE, reported in detail elsewhere (26), we addressed the following two questions:

1. Can substantial clot lysis, angiographically demonstrated, be achieved immediately after treatment with a 2-hr *peripheral intravenous* infusion of 50 mg of rt-PA followed, if necessary, by an additional 4-hr infusion of 40 mg of rt-PA?
2. Can rt-PA be administered safely (i.e., without major bleeding complications) to a select group of patients with acute PE?

This open-label study of rt-PA was designed to evaluate short-term efficacy and safety rather than to assess the possible long-term benefit of acutely administered rt-PA.

Patient Selection and Characteristics

The study population included adults with angiographically documented PE in a segmental or more proximal pulmonary artery within 5 days of the onset of symptoms or signs. Exclusion criteria were similar to those of the UPET except that patients could have undergone operation 7 (rather than 10) days earlier. For both UPET and our study, there was no upper age limit for enrollment, and patients with cancer were not excluded.

Of the 30 patients entered into the protocol, eight had undergone surgical treatment (four had received coronary artery bypass grafting). Their average age was 56 years and, prior to treatment, average pulmonary artery pressure was 35/14 (21) mm Hg.

Infusion of rt-PA

As soon as acute PE was documented angiographically, 50 mg of rt-PA (Activase®, supplied by Genentech, Inc.) was infused through a peripheral vein over 2 hours (25 mg/hr) (Figure 1). Pulmonary angiography was repeated

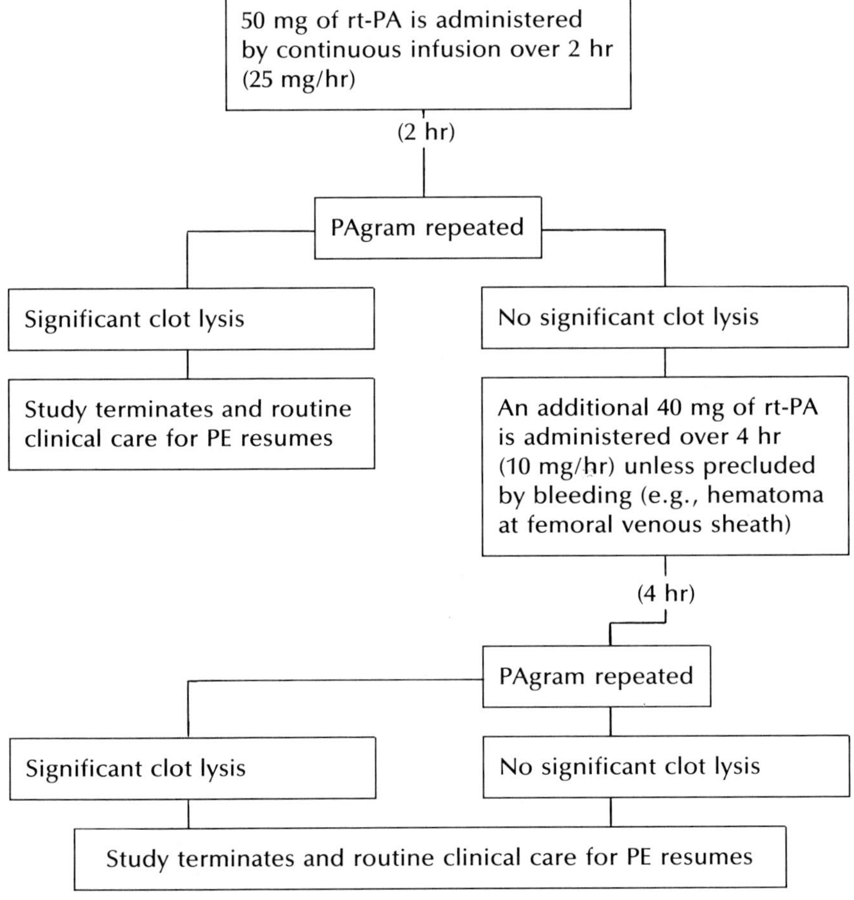

Figure 1   Steps in the rt-PA study protocol. PAgram = pulmonary angiogram; PE = pulmonary embolism.

immediately after the rt-PA infusion. If significant clot lysis was noted, the study was terminated and routine clinical care (usually including anticoagulation with heparin) was provided. If no significant clot lysis could be demonstrated, an additional 40 mg of rt-PA was administered over the next 4 hr (10 mg/hr), and a third pulmonary angiogram was obtained. When routine clinical care resumed, decisions regarding followup therapy with heparin, coumadin, or inferior vena caval interruption were made by the primary physician and were no longer part of the study protocol.

Assessment of Pulmonary Angiograms

Sets of pulmonary angiograms were coded and presented to a panel of six investigators for analysis. By means of blinded consensus reading, angiograms were first assessed *qualitatively* in terms of the extent of pulmonary artery thrombus (i.e., marked, moderate, slight, or unchanged). The same sets of angiograms were then assessed *quantitatively,* based on the scoring system used in the UPET (12). According to this system, a score of 0 represents no clot and the maximal score of 9 represents massive PE. Scores of 1 to 3 represent medium-sized PE, generally involving one lobe; scores of 3 to 7 represent large PE, generally involving two lobes; and scores of 7 to 9 represent massive PE, involving the entire lung.

Success in Clot Lysis

Overall, 28 of 30 patients had angiographic evidence of clot lysis after treatment with rt-PA [13 completed the study in 2 hr (Figure 2) and 17 remained in the study for 6 hr (Figures 3 and 4)]. Qualitative improvement as defined above was marked or moderate in 83% of patients. With regard to the quantitative scoring, the pretreatment angiographic score averaged 6.1, with improvement to 4.7 after 2 hr and further improvement to 3.2 after 6 hr (p < 0.001) (Figure 5), a 48% improvement.

Selective pulmonary angiography, as performed in this study, allowed only partial assessment of the pulmonary vasculature. However, lung scanning performed before and after rt-PA therapy in many of the patients indicated marked improvement in pulmonary perfusion after treatment (Figure 6) (27). Average pulmonary artery pressures decreased significantly after rt-PA therapy, from 35/14 ($\overline{21}$) to 30/13 ($\overline{18}$) mm Hg (p = 0.003). Among the patients with pulmonary hypertension, i.e., whose pulmonary artery mean pressure exceeded 17 mm Hg, the average pressure decreased from 39/16 ($\overline{24}$) to 32/14 ($\overline{20}$) mm Hg (p = 0.001). In some patients, right ventricular dysfunction and tricuspid regurgitation were documented with Doppler echocardiography prior to treatment and resolved rapidly after rt-PA therapy (Figure 7) (28). Plasma fibrinogen levels, measured using the sodium sulfite precipitation method of Rampling and Gaffney (29), decreased 37%, from an average of 351 mg/dl before treatment with rt-PA to 250 mg/dl after 2 hr and to 215 mg/dl after 6 hr of treatment (p < 0.001).

Complications of Therapy

Except for one patient, rt-PA therapy was tolerated without major complications, although the majority of the patients experienced superficial oozing from venipuncture or arterial puncture sites that was readily controlled with manual pressure and pressure dressings. The development of groin hematomas appeared to correlate with failure to cannulate the femoral vein percutaneously on the first attempt. Therapy was interrupted in five instances because of hematomas at the femoral venous catheter site: twice after 50 mg, twice after 80 mg, and once after 85 mg of an intended 90 mg dose of rt-PA. The single patient who had a major hemorrhagic complication had received 50 mg of rt-PA on the eighth day after coronary artery bypass surgery. Fifteen hours after treatment with rt-PA, emergency bedside drainage of the pericardial space was necessary, resulting in the evacuation of 500 ml of bloody fluid. After this experience, we modified the study protocol to exclude patients who have undergone open heart surgery until at least 3 weeks after the operation unless the PE is judged to be life-threatening.

rt-PA Compared With Other Modalities to Treat Acute PE

Although our open-label study was not intended to compare rt-PA infusion with conventional heparin therapy or with SK or UK infusion, the course of PE in patients treated with rt-PA did appear to differ substantially from that observed in patients treated with heparin or UK. In Phase I of UPET, pulmonary angiography was repeated approximately 24 hr after the initiation of therapy. Only 4% of the heparin-treated patients showed moderate or marked improvement, judged qualitatively, compared with 42% of the UK-treated patients. In our study with rt-PA, 83% showed evidence of moderate or marked qualitative improvement after only 2 or 6 hr. The percent improvement in quantitative score was 45% among the UK-treated patients over a 24-hr period and 48% among the rt-PA-treated patients over a 2- or 6-hr period.

The pretreatment perfusion defects on lung scanning appeared more extensive in the patients who received rt-PA than in the UPET patients, comprising 34% and 26% of the entire lung fields, respectively. In addition,

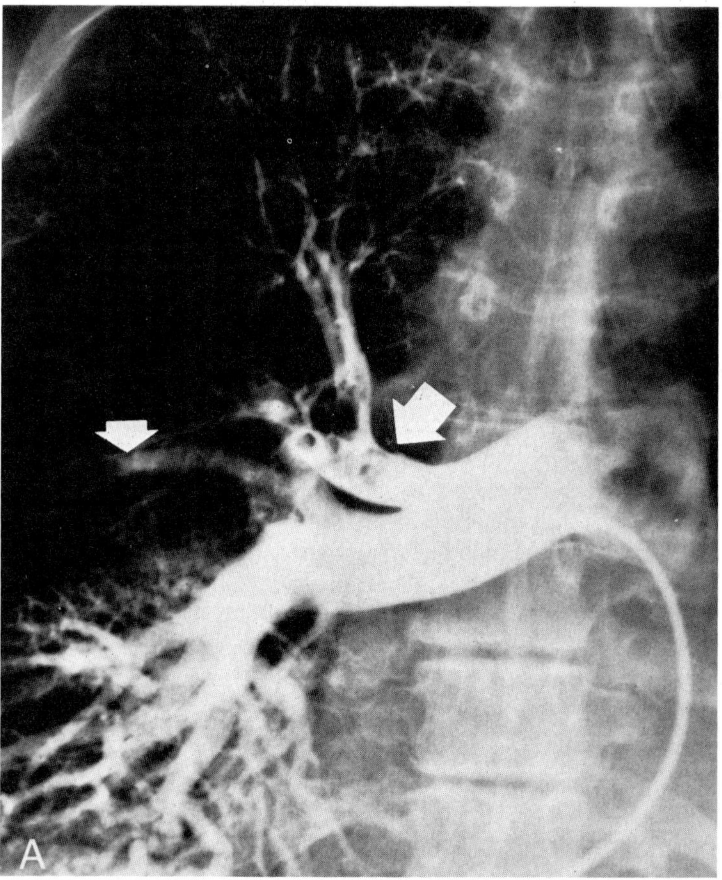

Figure 2A   Right anterior oblique pulmonary angiogram showing a large embolus in the right main pulmonary artery (arrows) in a 70-year-old woman who had undergone an ovarian carcinoma debulking operation 12 days previously.

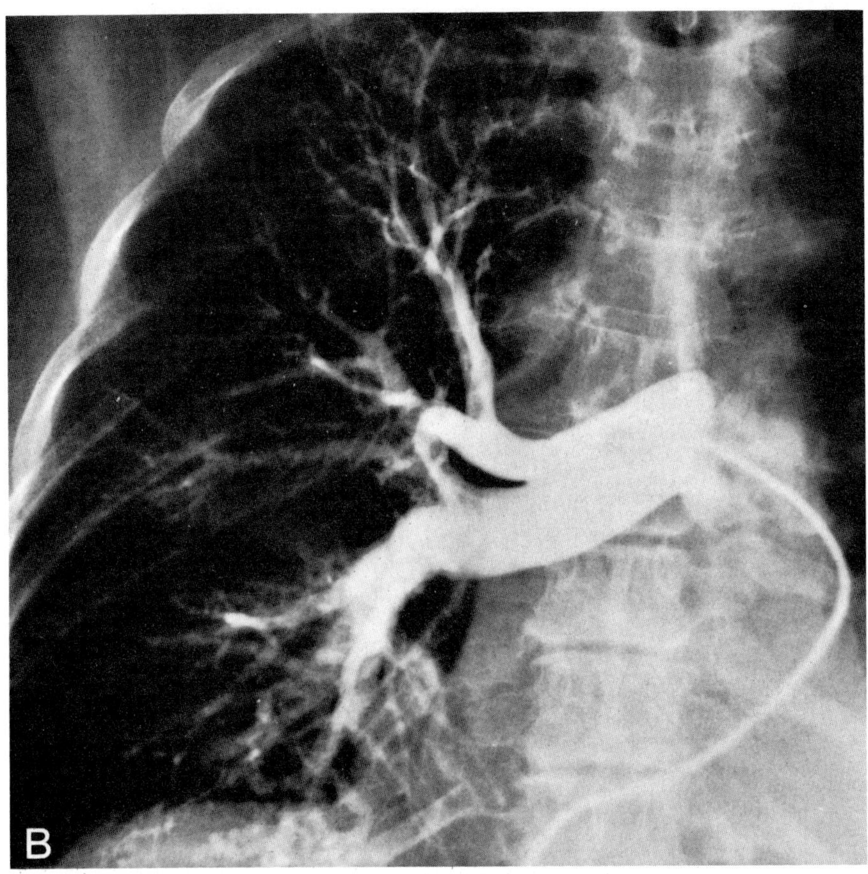

Figure 2B   After 2 hr of continuous infusion of rt-PA (50 mg), there is marked resolution of thrombi, with only a small amount of residual thrombus in segmental branches.

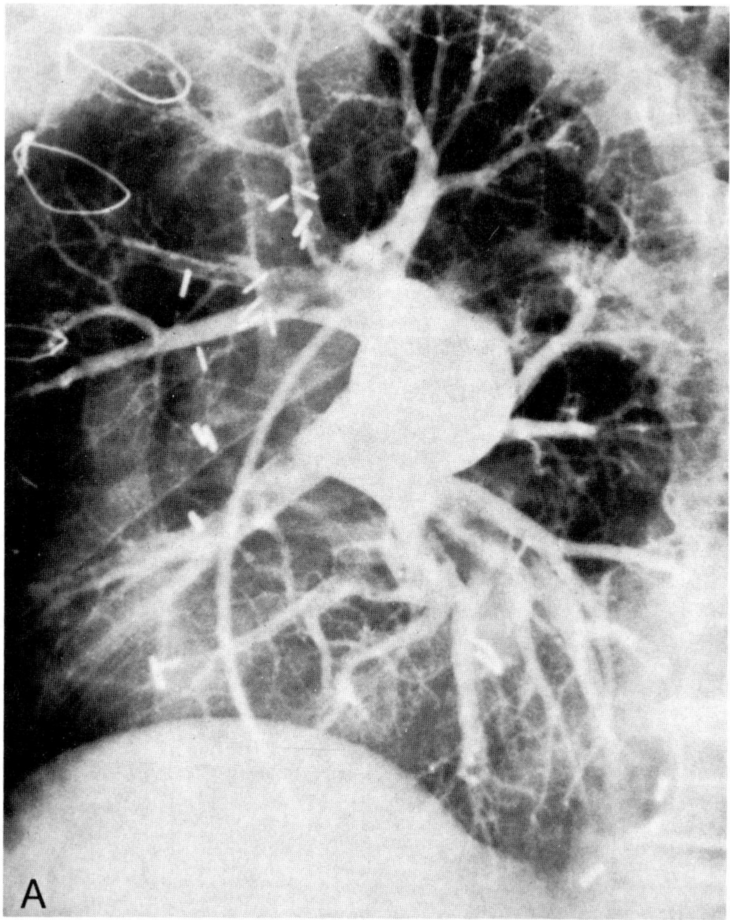

Figure 3A   Right posterior oblique pulmonary angiogram showing multiple emboli in the upper right, middle, and lower lung lobes in a 72-year-old man who had undergone coronary bypass grafting 12 days before.

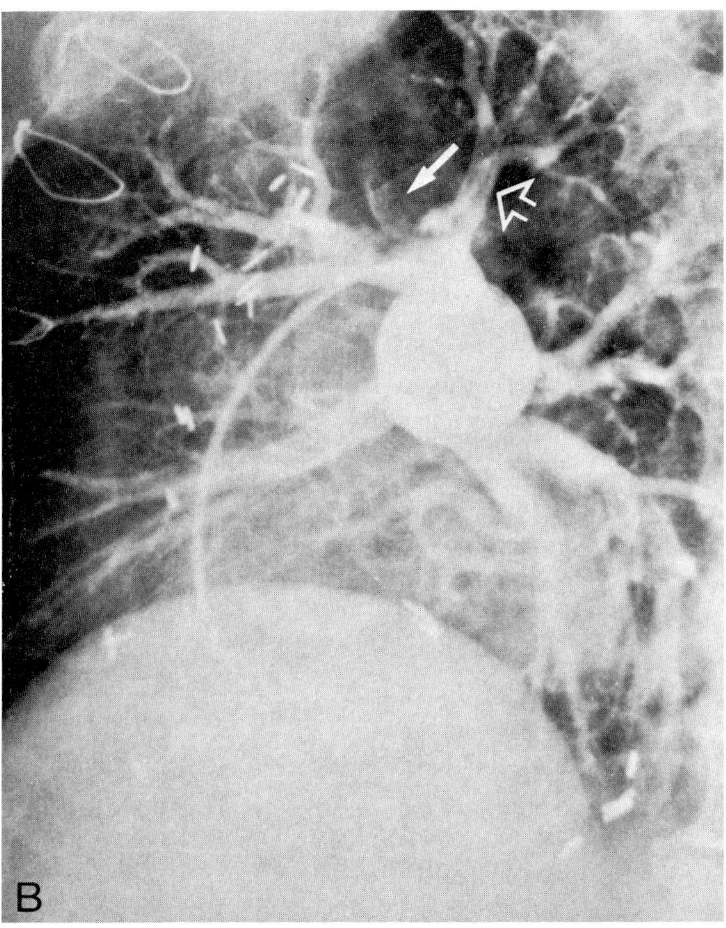

Figure 3B   After 2 hr of rt-PA infusion (50 mg), emboli in the anterior segment of the right upper, middle, and lower lobes have partially resolved. However, the apical segment of the right upper lobe is now completely occluded (closed arrow), and more thrombus is evident in the posterior segment of the right upper lobe (open arrow).

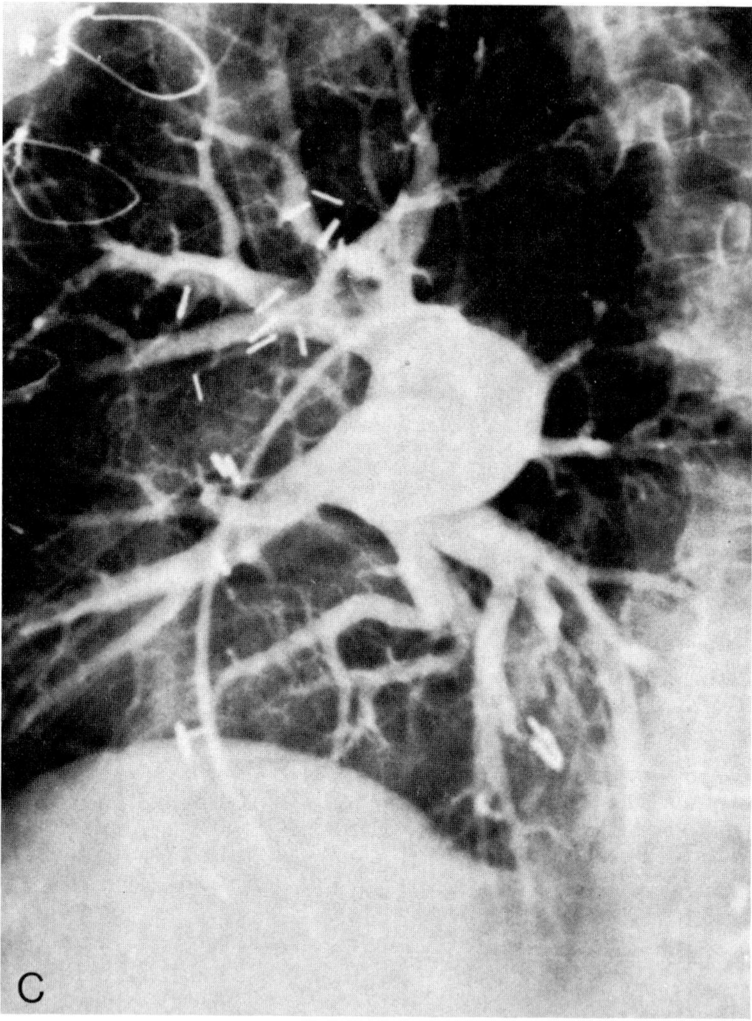

Figure 3C   After an additional 40 mg of rt-PA was infused over 4 hr (total dose =
90 mg over 6 hr), further resolution of emboli was evident in all areas and led to
reperfusion of the right upper lobe.

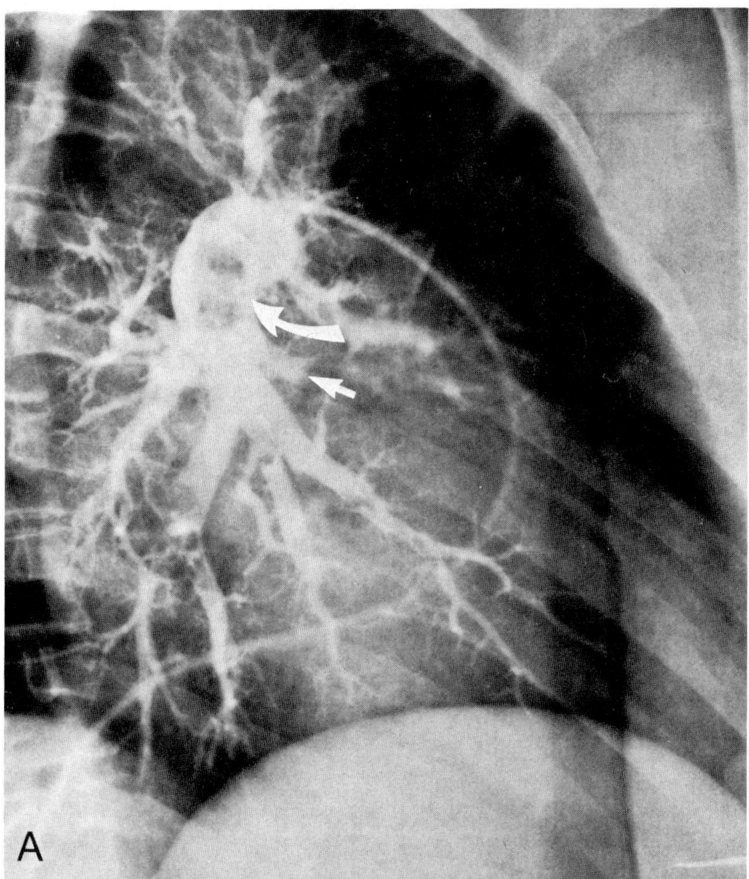

Figure 4A   Left posterior oblique pulmonary angiogram showing large thrombus in the left main pulmonary artery (curved arrow) and in multiple branches of the upper and lower lobes of a 30-year-old man with acute lymphoblastic leukemia in remission. There is a complete occlusion of the artery that supplies the lingula (straight arrow).

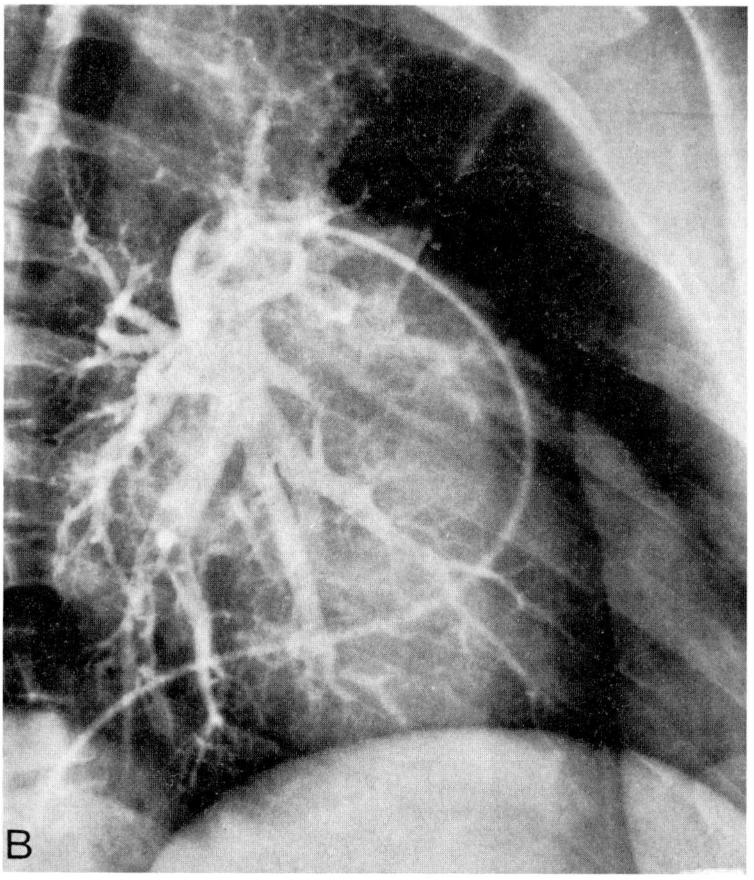

Figure 4B   After 2 hr of rt-PA infusion (50 mg), there is no significant improvement overall.

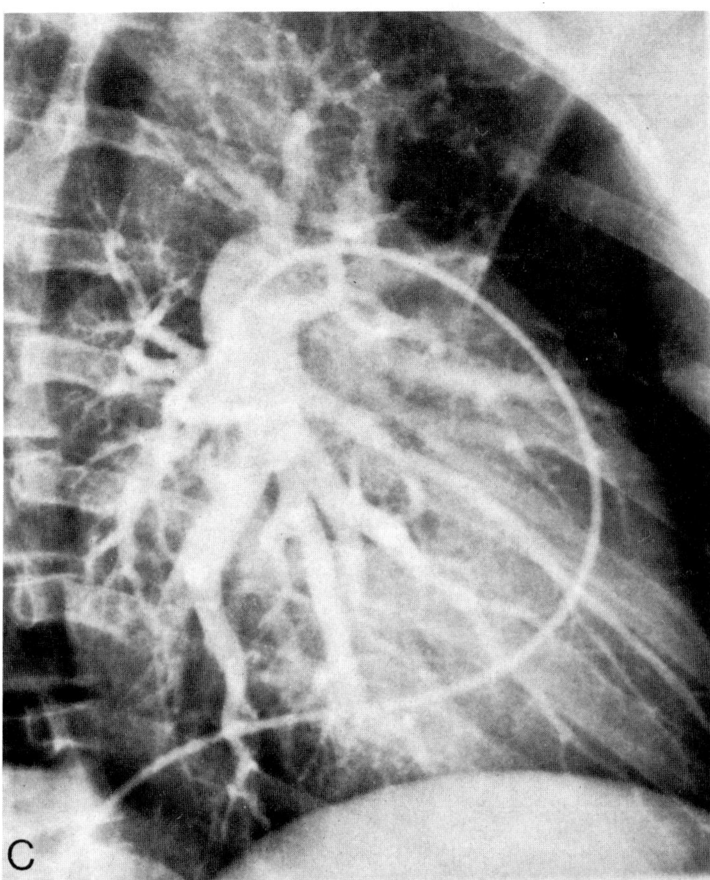

Figure 4C After an additional 40 mg of rt-PA was infused over 4 hr (total dose =
90 mg over 6 hr), there is complete resolution of the embolus in the main pulmonary
artery and upper lobe branches. There is improvement in the lower lobe branches,
although not complete resolution. The artery supplying the lingula is now patent.

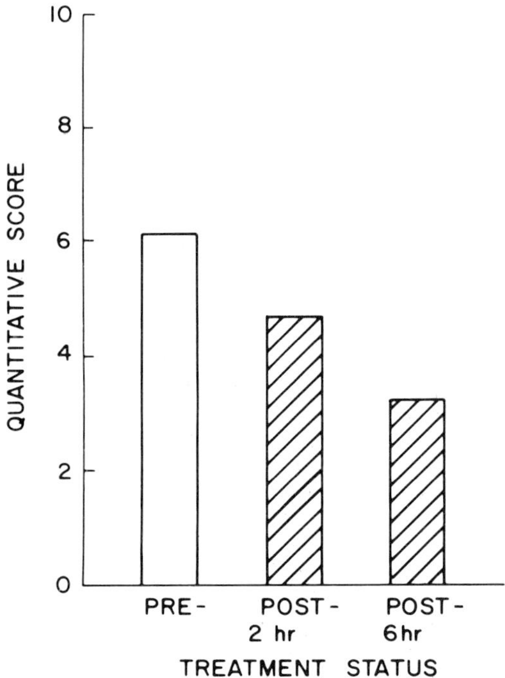

Figure 5   Quantitative analysis of the pulmonary angiogram before and after rt-PA treatment. (See text for explanation of scoring system.)

normalization of pulmonary perfusion on lung scans appeared to be more rapid in the rt-PA-treated patients compared with the UK-treated patients in UPET (27). The improvement in perfusion 1 day after rt-PA therapy was 58% using the UPET scoring method. By comparison, in the UPET trial there was a 24% improvement in perfusion after 24 hr of UK (and a 7% improvement with heparin) ($p < 0.001$).

Because rt-PA is only relatively fibrin-selective, it is not surprising that there was some reduction in plasma fibrinogen levels and that superficial oozing occurred at recent venipuncture sites or sites of arterial blood gas measurement (30). Nevertheless, our rate of major bleeding complications (3%) was lower than that seen among the UK-treated patients in either Phase I (27%) or Phase II (12%) of UPET (12,14). The 37% reduction in fibrinogen levels that we observed is consistent with findings among patients with myocardial infarction who received similar doses (31–34).

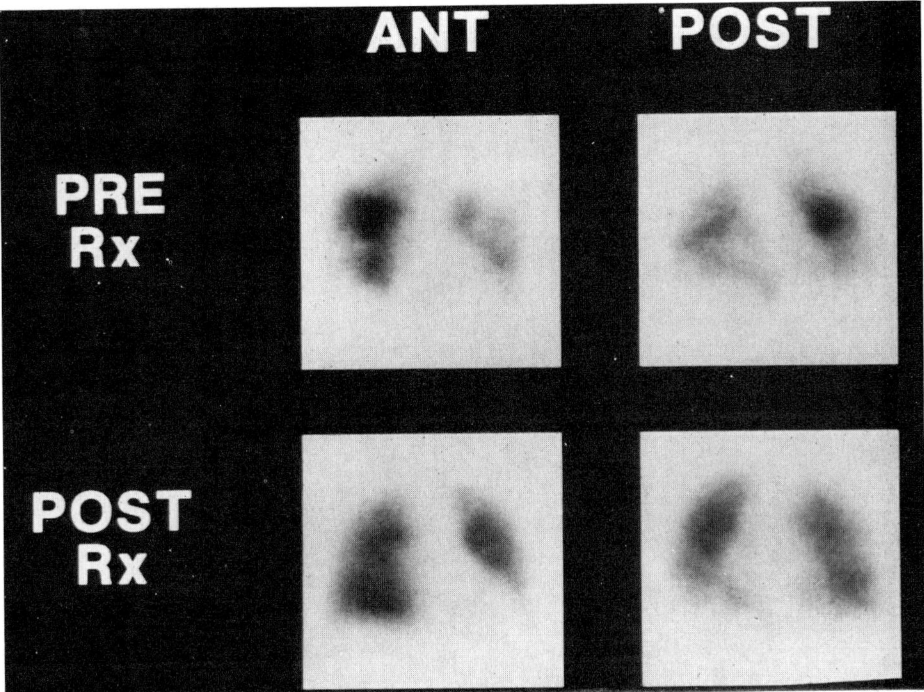

Figure 6 The anterior and posterior views of the pre-rt-PA therapy perfusion lung scan show massive pulmonary embolism in a 66-year-old man who presented with syncope. Except for a region in the midportion of the right lung, there is marked reduction and irregularity of perfusion in both lung fields. A lung scan performed 1 day after therapy with 90 mg of rt-PA shows nearly completely resolution of the defects. The only remaining perfusion defect is at the left base on the posterior view. ANT = anterior; POST = posterior. (Courtesy of J. Anthony Parker, M.D., Ph.D.)

Future Perspectives on rt-PA Therapy for Acute PE

Further studies are needed to determine under what circumstances the combination of rt-PA followed by heparin might be superior to standard heparin/ warfarin anticoagulation or treatment with a first-generation thrombolytic agent (i.e., UK or SK) followed by anticoagulation. Two separate small trials, one Canadian and one American, will utilize followup lung scanning and pulmonary angiography, respectively, to assess radiological improvement among patients assigned randomly to either rt-PA or anticoagulation therapy.

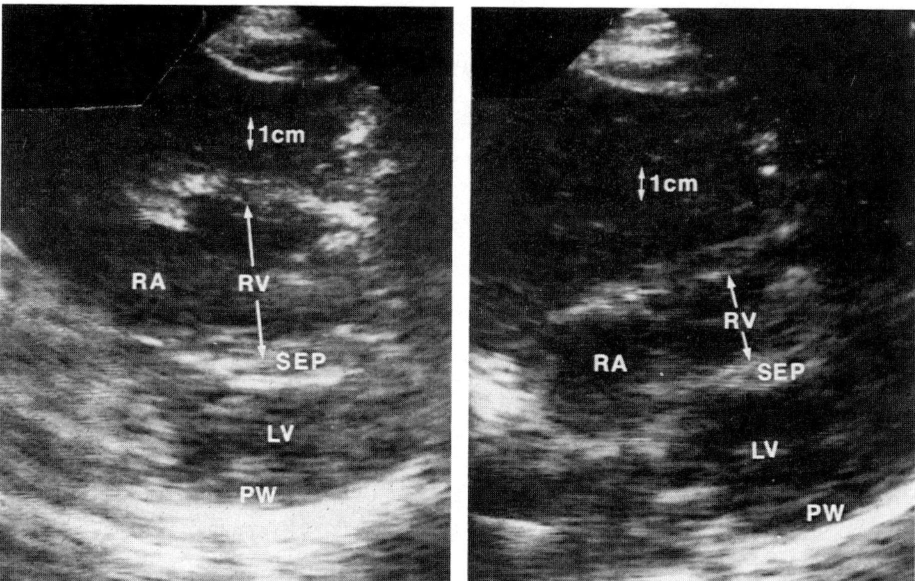

Figure 7   Subcostal two-dimensional echocardiogram of the patient (whose lung scan was presented in Figure 6) before (left) and after (right) rt-PA treatment. Prior to rt-PA therapy, the right ventricle was markedly dilated and measured 6.0 cm. In real time, the right ventricular contraction pattern was very hypokinetic. The Doppler echocardiographic examination demonstrated severe tricuspid regurgitation. After rt-PA therapy, the ventricular size normalized (2.4 cm). Furthermore, in real time, the right ventricular contraction pattern became normal and tricuspid regurgitation could no longer be detected by Doppler examination. RA = right atrium; RV = right ventricle; SEP = septum; LV = left ventricle; PW = posterior wall; 1 cm = 1 centimeter. (Courtesy of Patricia Come, M.D.)

At present, the clinical benefit of rt-PA therapy in acute PE appears most evident among patients with massive PE who have acute pulmonary hypertension and right ventricular dilation and dysfunction. In this group, the potential advantages of rt-PA appear to include lysis of large pulmonary arterial clots on serial angiograms and lung scans, leading to rapid reduction of abnormally elevated right heart pressures and restoration of normal right ventricular function. Although studies comparing rt-PA with other lytic agents and with anticoagulation alone are lacking, the encouraging results to date suggest that rt-PA will eventually become standard therapy for patients with massive PE who do not have contraindications to lytic treatment. It is more difficult to predict the eventual role of rt-PA therapy for patients with medium-sized or submassive PE. These patients for the most part currently receive heparin/ warfarin anticoagulation as standard treatment, without lytic therapy. Use of rt-PA in these patients will occur if a multicentered cooperative trial demonstrates clinically significant long-term benefit in addition to radiological improvement. A large-scale trial of rt-PA versus standard anticoagulation would be timely to test the folowing hypotheses related to clinical outcome that have been formulated during treatment of PE with open-label rt-PA: 1) rt-PA treatment can reduce the recurrence rate of PE; 2) rt-PA treatment can more often permanently restore to normal right ventricular function and pulmonary artery pressure. We believe that such a trial is worthwhile to place this new, very promising therapy in its most proper perspective.

REFERENCES

1. Goldhaber SZ, Hennekens CH: Time trends in hospital mortality and diagnosis of pulmonary embolism. Am Heart J 104:305–306, 1982.
2. Wessler S: *Prevention of Venous Thromboembolism: Rationale, Practice, and Problems*, NIH 1986 Consensus Development Conference on Prevention of Venous Thrombosis and Pulmonary Embolism, National Institutes of Health, Bethesda, Maryland, 1986.
3. Dalen JE, Banas JS, Brooks HC, et al: Resolution rate of acute pulmonary embolism in man. N Engl J Med 280:1194, 1969.
4. Tow DE, Wagner NH Jr: Recovery of pulmonary artery flow in patients with pulmonary embolism. N Engl J Med 276:1053, 1967.
5. Urokinase Pulmonary Embolism Trial, Phase 1 Results. JAMA 214:2163, 1970.
6. Hirsh J, McDonald IG, Hale GA, et al: Comparison of the effects of streptokinase and heparin the early rate of resolution of major pulmonary embolism. Can Med Assoc J 104:488–491, 1971.
7. Miller GAH, Sutton GC, Kerr IH, et al: Comparison of streptokinase and heparin in the treatment of isolated acute massive pulmonary embolism. Br Med J 2:681–684, 1971.
8. Tibbutt DA, Davies JA, Anderson JA, et al: Comparison by controlled clinical trial of streptokinase and heparin in the treatment of life-threatening pulmonary embolism. Br Med J 2:343–347, 1974.
9. Ly B, Arnesen H, Eie H, Hol R: A controlled clinical trial of streptokinase and heparin in the treatment of major pulmonary embolism. Acta Med Scand 203: 465–470, 1978.
10. Hoagland PM: Massive pulmonary embolism. In *Pulmonary Embolism and Deep Venous Thrombosis*, Goldhaber SZ, Ed., WB Saunders, Philadelphia, 1985, pp. 179–208.

11. Freiman JA, Chalmers TC, Smith H, et al: The importance of beta, the type II error and sample size in the design and interpretation of the randomized control trial. Survey of 71 "negative" trials. N Engl J Med 299:690, 1978.

12. The Urokinase Pulmonary Embolism Trial: A national cooperative study. Circulation 47(suppl II):II-1–II-108, 1973.

13. Sharma GVRK, Burleson VA, Sasahara AA: Effect of thrombolytic therapy on pulmonary capillary blood volume in patients with pulmonary embolism. N Engl J Med 303:842–945, 1980.

14. Urokinase Pulmonary Embolism Trial Group: Urokinase-streptokinase embolism trial: Phase 2 results. JAMA 229:1606–1613, 1974.

15. Thrombolytic therapy in thrombosis: A National Institutes of Health Consensus Development Conference. Ann Intern Med 93:141, 1980.

16. Gruppo Italiano Per Lo Studio Della Streptochinasi Nell'Infarto Miocardico (GISSI): Effectiveness of intravenous thrombolytic treatment in acute myocardial infarction. Lancet 1:397–402, 1986.

17. Yusuf S, Collins R, Peto R, et al: Intravenous and intracoronary fibrinolytic therapy in acute myocardial infarction: Overview of results on mortality, reinfarction, and side-effects from 33 randomised controlled trials. Eur Heart J 6:556–585, 1985.

18. Pennica D, Holmes WE, Kohr WJ, Harkins RN, Vehar GA, Ward CA, Bennett WF, Yelverton E, Seeburg PH, Heyneker HL, Goeddel DV: Cloning and expression of human tissue-type plasminogen activator cDNA in *E. coli*. Nature 301:214–221, 1983.

19. Korninger C, Matsuo O, Suy R, Stassen JM, Collen D: Thrombolysis with human extrinsic (tissue-type) plasminogen activator in dogs with femoral vein thrombosis. J Clin Invest 69:573–580, 1982.

20. Collen D, Stassen JM, Verstraete M: Thrombolysis with human extrinsic (tissue-type) plasminogen activator in rabbits with experimental jugular vein thrombosis. Effect of molecular form and dose of activator, age of the thrombus, and route of administration. J Clin Invest 71:368–376, 1983.

21. Agnelli G, Buchanan MR, Fernandez F, Boneu R, Van Ryn J, Hirsh J, Collen D: A comparison of the thrombolytic and hemorrhagic effects of tissue-type plasminogen activator and streptokinase in rabbits. Circulation 72:178–182, 1985.

22. Matsuo O, Rijken DC, Collen D: Thrombolysis by human tissue plasminogen activator and urokinase in rabbits with experimental pulmonary embolus. Nature 291:590–591, 1981.

23. Weimar W, Stibbe J, van Seyen AJ, Billiau A, DeSomer P, Collen D: Specific lysis of an iliofemoral thrombus by administration of extrinsic (tissue-type) plasminogen activator. Lancet 2:1018–1020, 1981.

24. Turpie AGG, Jay RM, Carter CJ, Hirsh J: A randomized trial of recombinant tissue plasminogen activator for the treatment of proximal deep vein thrombosis. Circulation 72(abstr):III-193, 1985.

25. Bounameaux H, Vermylen J, Collen D: Thrombolytic treatment with recombi-
     nant tissue-type plasminogen activator in a patient with massive pulmonary
     embolism. Ann Intern Med 103:64–66, 1985.
26. Goldhaber SZ, Vaughan DE, Markis JE, Selwyn AP, Meyerovitz ME, Loscalzo
     J, Kim DS, Kessler CM, Dawley DL, Sharma GVRK, Sasahara A, Grossbard
     EB, Braunwald E: Acute pulmonary embolism treated with tissue plasminogen
     activator. Lancet 2:886–889, 1986.
27. Markis JE, Goldhaber SZ, Kim DS, Palla A, Parker JA, Braunwald E: Early
     improved pulmonary perfusion after intravenous recombinant tissue plasminogen
     activator for acute pulmonary embolism. Circulation 74(abstr):II-127, 1986.
28. Come PC, Markis JE: Reversal of right ventricular dysfunction in patients after
     intravenous tissue plasminogen activator for acute pulmonary embolism. JACC
     9(abstr): in press, 1987.
29. Rampling MW, Gaffney PJ: The sulphite precipitation method for fibrinogen
     measurement: its use on small samples in the presence of fibrinogen degradation
     products. Clin Chim Acta 67:43–52, 1976.
30. Sobel BE, Gross RW, Robison AK: Thrombolysis, clot selectivity, and kinetics.
     Circulation 70:160–164, 1984.
31. Williams DO: Intravenous recombinant tissue type plasminogen activator (rt-
     PA) in acute myocardial infarction: a report from the NHLBI Thrombolysis in
     Myocardial Infarction (TIMI) trial. J Am Coll Cardiol 5(abstr):495, 1985.
32. Topol EJ, Bell WR, Weisfeldt ML: Coronary thrombolysis with recombinant
     tissue-type plasminogen activator. A hematologic and pharmacologic study. Ann
     Intern Med 103:837–843, 1985.
33. Owen J, Friedman KD, Berke AD, Grossman BA, Wilkins C, Powers ER:
     Fibrinogenolysis induced by tissue plasminogen activator and by streptokinase.
     Blood 66(abstr)(suppl I):325a, 1985.
34. Collen D, Bounameaux H, De Cock F, Lijnen HR, Verstraete M: Analysis of
     coagulation and fibrinolysis during intravenous infusion of recombinant human
     tissue-type plasminogen activator in patients with acute myocardial infarction.
     Circulation 73:511–517, 1986.

10

Thrombolysis with Recombinant Human Tissue-Type Plasminogen Activator in Patients with Peripheral Artery and Bypass Graft Thrombosis

Robert A. Graor and Barbara Risius
Cleveland Clinic
Cleveland, Ohio

I. INTRODUCTION

Thrombolysis using intraarterial streptokinase (SK) and urokinase (UK) has been successfully employed as a therapeutic alternative or adjuvant modality in the treatment of thrombosed peripheral arteries and bypass grafts (1–7). This treatment approach has achieved relatively slow acceptance, reflected in part by the misconceptions of lytic therapy, lack of definitive endpoints for efficacy, and durability of results, and by the risks associated with thrombolysis.

First-generation thrombolytic agents (SK and UK) activate the fibrinolytic system by converting both circulating and fibrin-bound plasminogen to plasmin, the proteolytic enzyme that digests fibrin. Despite alterations in dosage of thrombolytic agents, a systemic lytic state generally ensues, and this may predispose these patients to an increased risk of hemorrhage (7–9). Bleeding and antigenic reactions (predominantly with streptokinase) are relatively frequent with the intraarterial infusions of conventional fibrinolytic agents. These risks have often exceeded the risks associated with primary vascular repair. Therefore, the use of intraarterial infusions of thrombolytic agents mandates selection of patients who cannot otherwise be treated by surgical repair in a safer and more expeditious manner.

Initial experience with recombinant human tissue-type plasminogen activator (rt-PA) has provided evidence that this new second-generation thrombolytic agent has potential advantages over previously used agents (10–18). As this experience accumulates, data may provide evidence that properly selected patients will be better suited for initial treatment with rt-PA thrombolysis than for primary vascular surgical repair.

Prolonged infusions of rt-PA in patients with occluded thrombosed peripheral arteries and bypass grafts have provided preliminary information on the dose/time influence of this clot-selective agent on the constituents of the fibrinolytic system.

II. PATIENT SELECTION

Patients under consideration for primary vascular surgical repair were considered candidates for administration of fibrinolytic agents. Following complete examination, segmental Doppler pressures and plethysmography recordings were obtained to establish the hemodynamic significance of the occlusion and provide a baseline for comparison following thrombus lysis. Angiographic documentation of the occluded thromboembolism was obtained before the administration of the fibrinolytic agent. This established the site and the extent of involvement, and aided in deciding whether the occlusion was amenable to thrombolytic therapy. It also established a baseline from which results of thrombolysis can be assessed (Figure 1).

Exclusion criteria were: 1) a history of a bleeding diathesis, 2) a central nervous system tumor, abscess, arteriovenous malformation, aneurysm, or previous central nervous system bleeding (patients who had had ischemic cerebral infarctions of embolic or thrombotic nature underwent treatment if at least 1 year had elapsed from the time of the most recent neurological change), 3) a history of internal bleeding within the previous 4 weeks, unless the bleeding originated from a gastric ulcer and an endoscopic procedure had proven this to be healed, 4) a history of major surgery, intrathoracic or intraabdominal, within the preceding 21 days (patients undergoing vascular surgery within the preceding 21 days were not necessarily excluded), 5) a history of clinically significant hepatic disease causing alterations in hemostatic function, 6) the presence of fewer than 70,000 platelets, or 70,000–100,000 platelets with an abnormal bleeding time, and 7) pregnancy.

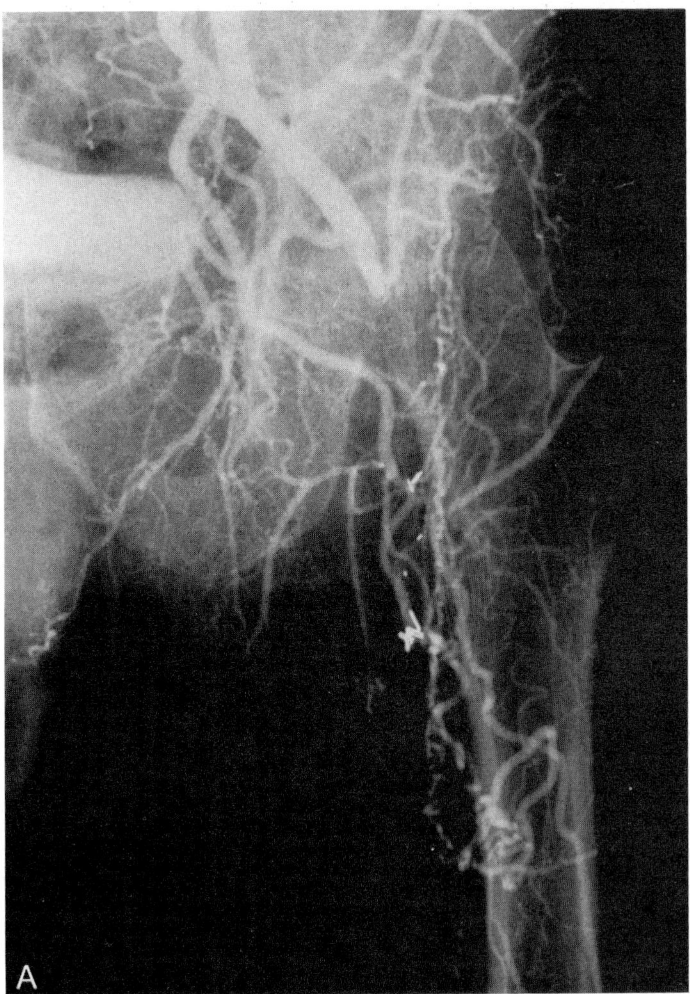

Figure 1 (A–C) Left femoral arteriogram showing occlusion of the distal common femoral artery in a 47-year-old man with a prior history of a common femoral endarterectomy with patch angioplasty and patch angioplasty of the distal superficial femoral artery. The patient presents with left-leg ischemia of 4 days' duration. Multiple collaterals reconstitute a distal superficial femoral artery with subsequent opacification of popliteal and tibial arteries which appear normal. (D, E) After 6 hr of rt-PA, complete thrombolysis reveals a false aneurysm at the common femoral patch angioplasty site.

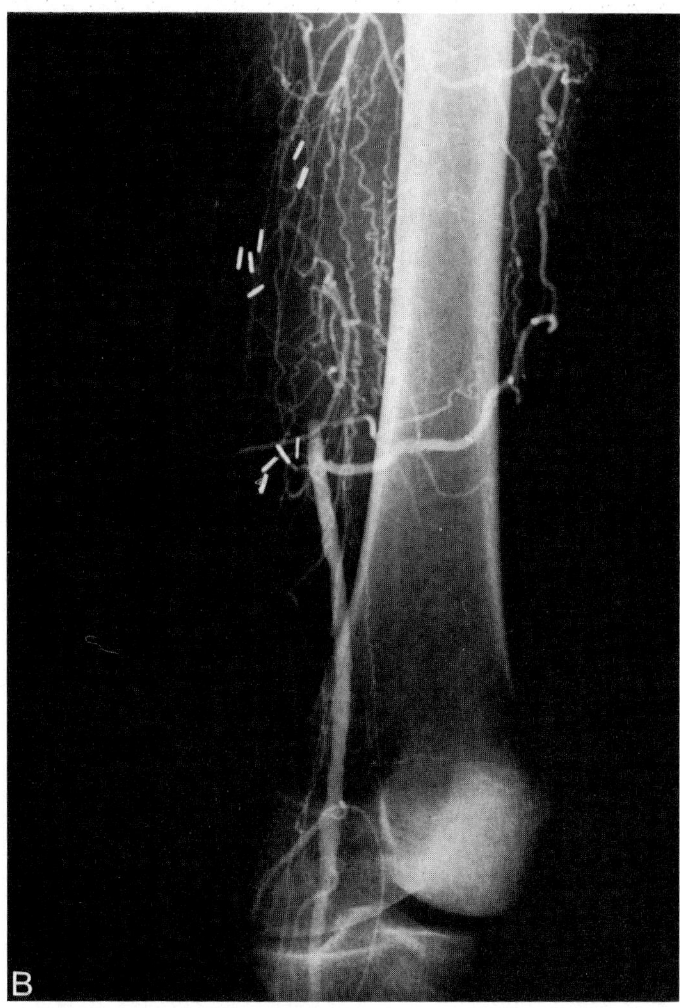

Figure 10.1 (Continued)

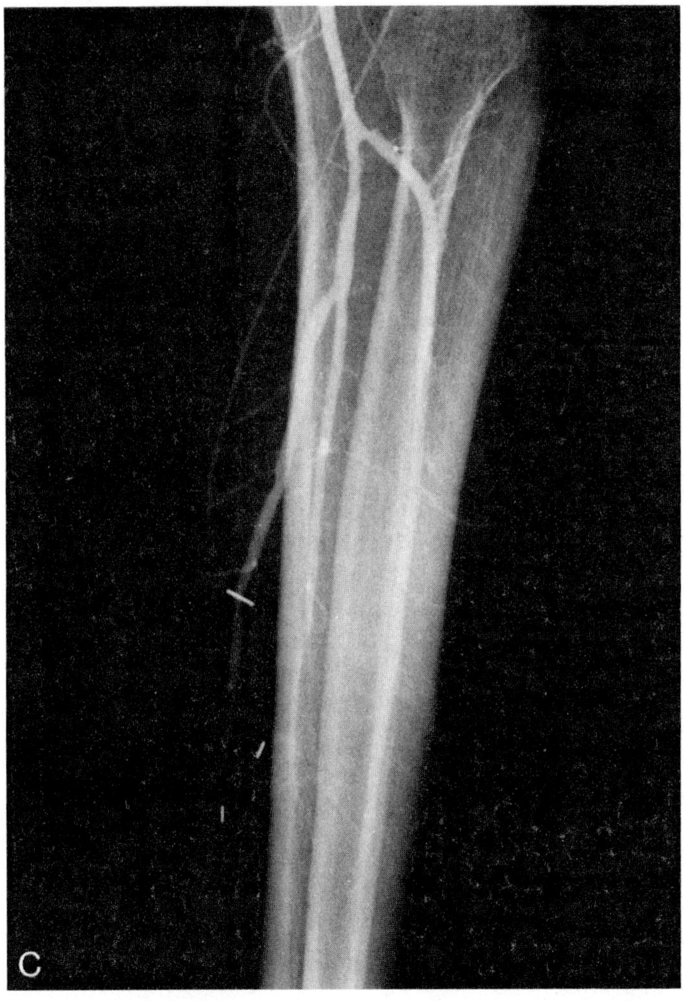

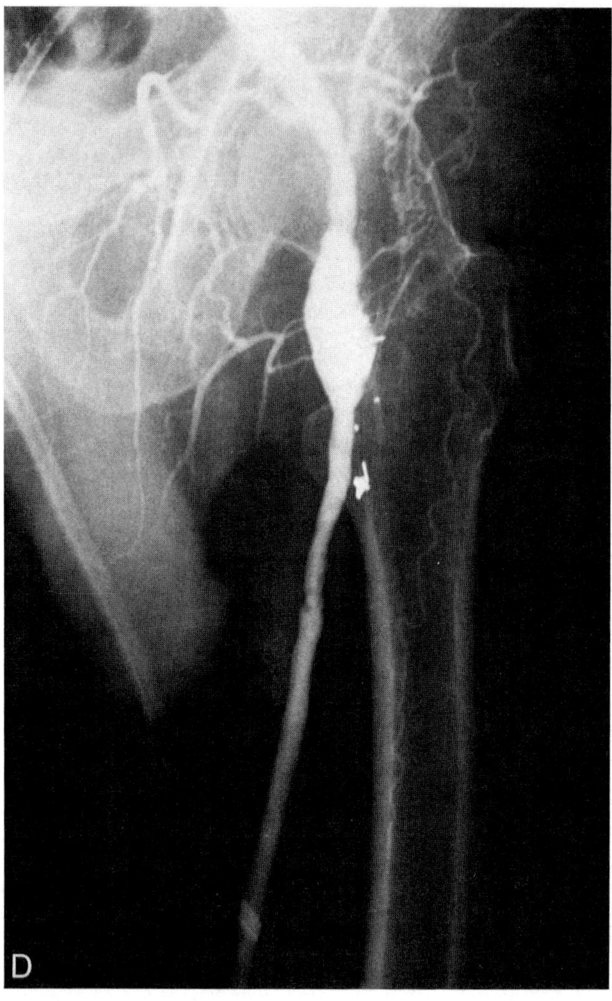

Figure 10.1 (Continued)

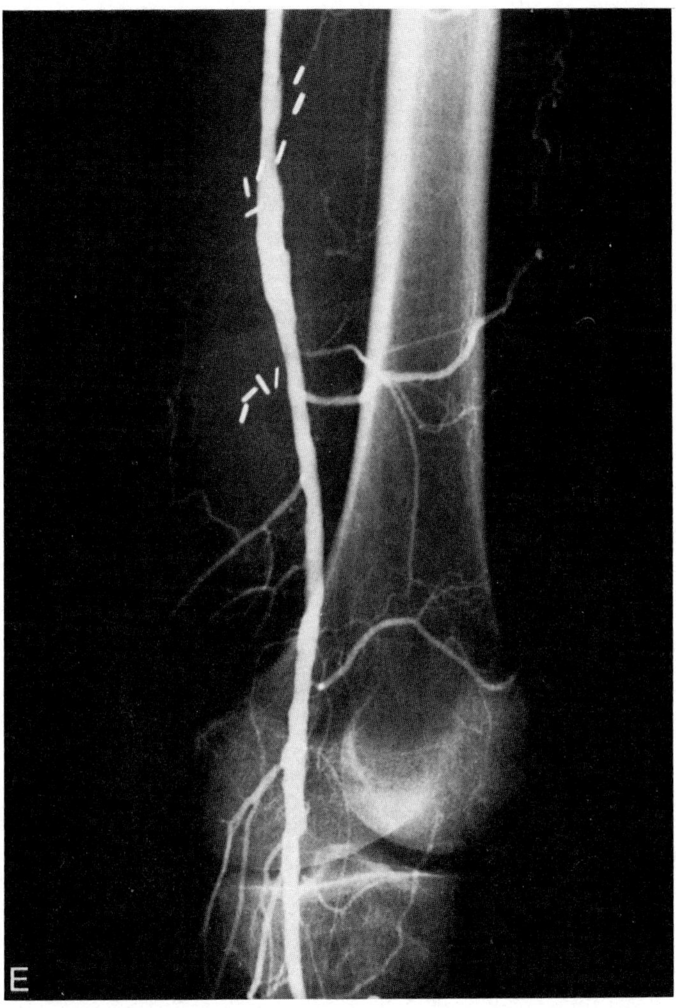

III. METHODS

Between October 1984 and June 1986, 55 patients with extremity ischemia secondary to thrombosed peripheral arteries or bypass grafts were treated with rt-PA (Table 1). Twenty-nine of 55 patients (53%) had prior vascular surgery involving the limb in which rt-PA was infused. Twenty-one of the 29 had bypass grafts, five of which were constructed in the same hospital stay during which rt-PA was infused. Four patients had incomplete thromboembolectomies immediately prior to rt-PA infusion (Figure 2).

rt-PA was infused at a dosage of 0.1 or 0.05 mg/kg/hr. The first 19 patients studied received the 0.1-mg/kg/hr dosage, and the remaining patients were alternately treated with 0.1 or 0.05 mg/kg/hr. The dosage schedule was changed because the initial high success rate of thrombus lysis suggested that a lower dosage might be equally effective and even more fibrinogen-sparing. Notwithstanding the alteration in dosage, other aspects of the protocol, such as infusion duration, endpoints, and the method of verification of thrombus lysis, remained unchanged.

rt-PA was infused through an angiographic catheter embedded into the thrombus. Infusion durations did not exceed 8 hr. Catheter entry points were chosen according to the location of the thrombus and were always in regions where the artery could be compressed manually.

Blood chemistries, complete blood count (including platelet count and differential white blood count), fibrinogen, fibrin(ogen) split products, plasminogen, α_2-antiplasmin, prothrombin time (PT), activated partial thromboplastin time (APTT), and thrombin time (TT) were measured before infusion and at 2, 4, 6, and 8 hr during the infusion and at 24 hr and at 30 days following infusion.

The PT and APTT results were obtained with thromboplastin C and actin (American Dade, Inc.) and the MLA-700 automated instrument. The fibrinogen was measured by the Clauss method (American Dade thrombin reagen) and by the sodium sulfite precipitation method. rt-PA antigen levels were determined by the enzyme-linked immunosorbin assay (ELISA) method. The TT was determined by human thrombin (Ortho Diagnostics). The plasminogen and α_2-antiplasmin values were measured by synthetic fluorogenic assay (American Dade Protopath). Fibrin(ogen) split products were measured by latex agglutination method (Thrombo Welco, Burroughs Wellcome, Inc.). Protamine paracoagulation of plasma was used to test for soluable fibrin products. Blood was collected from an indwelling central venous catheter placed before the initiation of rt-PA infusion in glass tubes on citrate or citrate containing aprotinin (Trasylol; Bayer) (final concentration 250 KIU/ml blood) or D-phenyl-alanyl-L-prolyl-L-arginine chloromethyl ketone · 2 HCl (PPACK) (400 mi-

Table 1   Patient Data and Characteristics
of Thrombotic or Embolic Occlusions in 55
Patients Treated with t-PA

Age	
Mean (yr)	58
Range (yr)	26–76
Male/female	38/17
Type of occlusion	
Arterial	28
thrombotic	16
embolic	12
Grafts	27
SVG[a]	12
PTFE[b]	12
Dacron	3
Age of occlusion (days)	
Mean	7.5
Range	1–26
Duration of infusions (hr)	
Mean	4.7
Range	1–8
Total dosage infused	
Group 1 (37) (mg)[c]	
mean	34.1
range	9–58
Group 2 (18) (mg)[d]	
mean	21.5
range	8.8–36

[a]Saphenous vein graft.
[b]Polytetrafluoroethylene.
[c]0.1 mg/kg/hr.
[d]0.05 mg/kg/hr.

cromolar stock in 0.01 NHCl) for inhibition of in vitro t-PA activity in samples collected. Tests of plasminogen and α_2-antiplasmin were either performed immediately with fresh plasma or with samples frozen for up to 12 hours at -70 degrees centigrade. All other tests were performed within 30 minutes of the venipuncture.

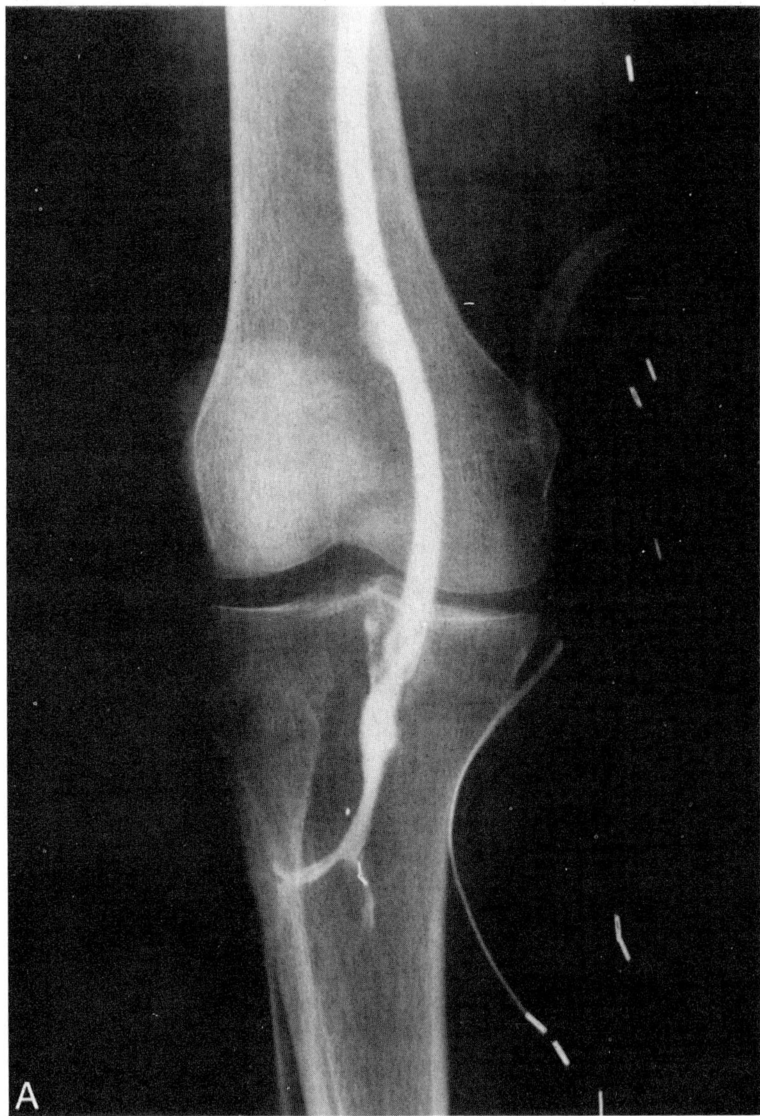

Figure 2   (A) A right femoral arteriogram following unsuccessful surgical throm-bectomy of a thrombosed femoropopliteal bypass graft demonstrates small residual thrombi within the graft and occlusion of all tibial arteries in a patient with 3 days of ischemic rest pain. (B, C) Following 2 hr of rt-PA infusion, there has been complete thrombus lysis in the anterior tibial artery establishing flow into the foot.

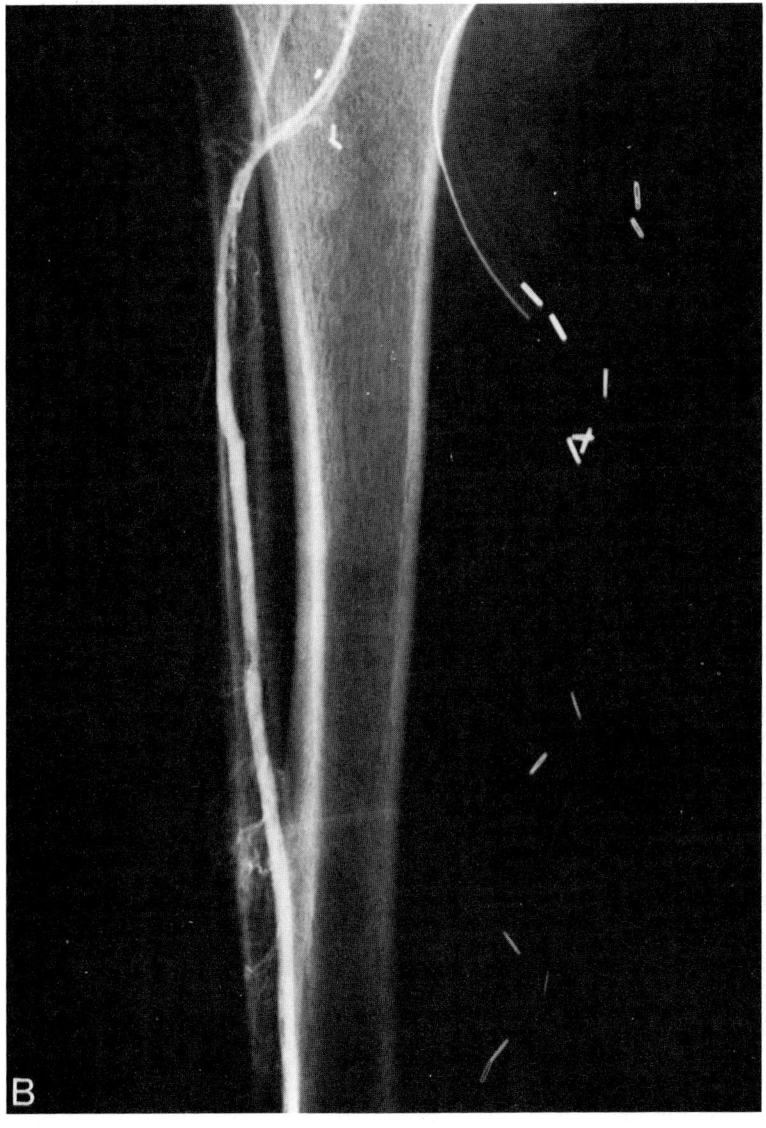

B

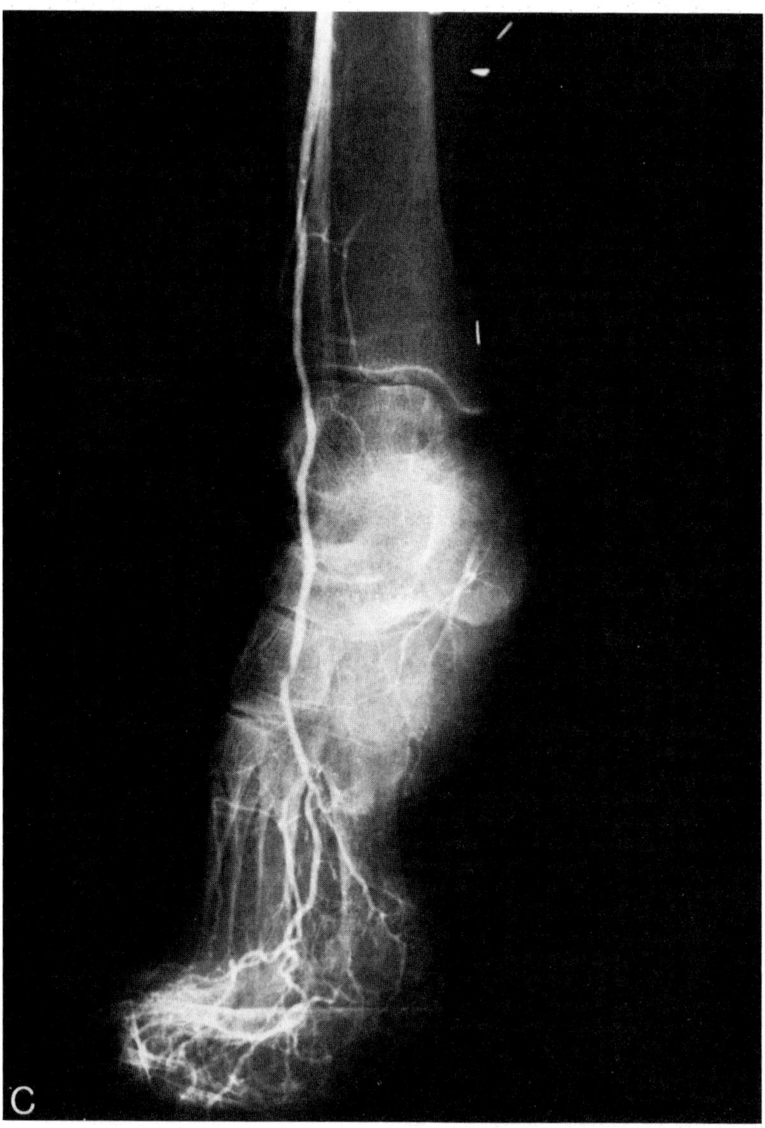

Figure 10.2 (Continued)

IV. RESULTS

Thrombolysis occurred in 51 of 55 patients (93%). There was no difference in the incidence of successful thrombus lysis between the 0.05- and 0.1-mg/kg/hr dosage groups. Four patients failed to achieved thrombolysis, two received the 0.05 dose, and two received the 0.1-mg/kg/hr dosage. Two patients had thrombosed femoropopliteal bypass grafts that could not be selectively catheterized. A third patient had an occluded, in situ, saphenous-vein femoropopliteal bypass graft that was obliterated due to a scarred tunnel near the popliteal artery (documented at the time of revision surgery). The fourth patient had partial thrombolysis revealing a distal radial artery aneurysm that was responsible for digital emboli. rt-PA was discontinued once the aneurysm was visualized in an attempt to prevent further emboli from occurring and avoid the need for surgical clipping. The hand remained viable.

Forty-eight of the 51 patients (94%) experienced angiographic as well as prolonged clinical benefit from thrombolysis. Three patients had successful thrombolysis but no clinical improvement due to severely atherosclerotic distal disease that precluded surgical repair or successful anticoagulation to maintain patency. No clinical deterioration resulted from attempted thrombus lysis in these three patients or in the four patients who did not achieve thrombus lysis angiographically. In the patients who were successfully treated, mean improvement in ankle-brachial ratios was 0.38 (range 0.10–0.82).

Secondary procedures (vascular surgery or balloon angioplasty) to maintain arterial or graft patency were required in 29 of 51 patients (57%). Fourteen of these patients required graft anastomotic revisions (11 distal and three proximal revisions), six patients had endarterectomies with patch angioplasty in the region of thrombolysis, and three patients required a new bypass entirely. In two patients an above-knee amputation was anticipated prior to thrombus lysis. One of these patients was converted to a below-knee amputation following profunda femoris artery thrombus lysis, and the second was converted to a transmetatarsal amputation following popliteal and tibial outflow thrombus lysis. One additional patient had a local revision of a transmetatarsal amputation and did not require a higher level of amputation to be performed. Balloon angioplasty was performed following thrombus lysis in three patients. Sixteen of 51 (31%) patients required anticoagulation to maintain vascular segment patency, and three (6%) additional patients required no further treatment.

rt-PA blood levels averaged 2.6 ng/ml before and after infusion (range 0–5.5 ng/ml) and 155.7 ng/ml (range 13.4–1000 ng/ml) during infusions. In patients treated with the 0.1-mg/kg/hr dosage and those receiving the 0.05-mg/kg/hr dose, the activator antigen levels averaged 232.4 ng/ml (range 73–1000 ng/ml) and 65.6 ng/ml (range 10–138 ng/ml), respectively.

Infusion of rt-PA resulted in α_2-antiplasmin changes illustrated in Figure 3. At 2 hr of infusion, the differences in α_2-antiplasmin between the 0.1- and 0.05-mg/kg/hr dosages achieved statistical significance ($p < 0.05$). No significant difference was seen at 4- and 6-hour values.

Figure 4 demonstrates differences in fibrinogen levels determined by the clottable method (Clauss) and sodium sulfite precipitation method at dosages of 0.05 and 0.1 mg/kg/hr.

Among the 37 patients receiving the 0.1-mg/kg/hr dosage, plasminogen levels decreased an average of 75%. In none was there a complete depletion of circulating plasminogen. Among patients treated with the 0.05-

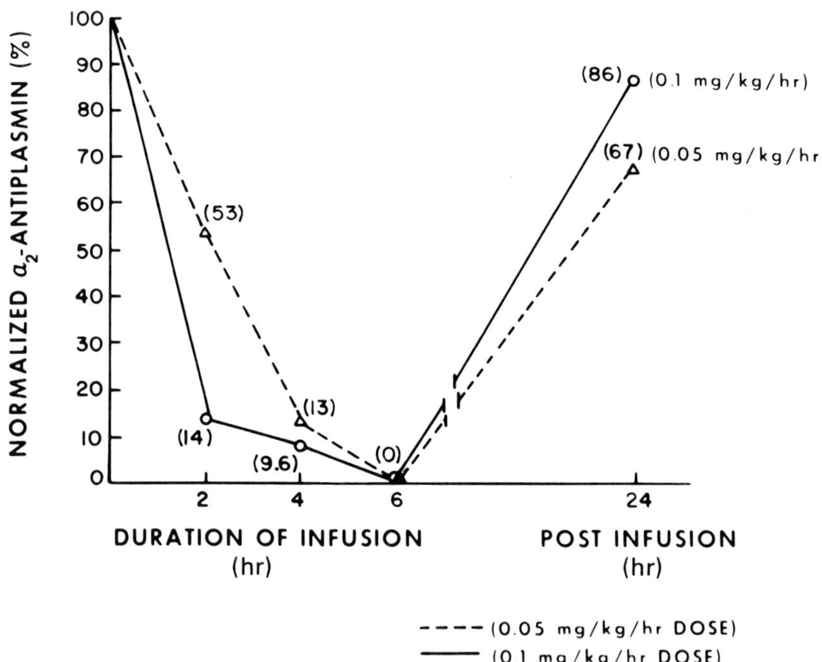

Figure 3   Comparative mean normalized fibrinogen values in rt-PA-treated patients receiving the 0.1-mg/kg/hr dosage (n = 37) and the 0.05-mg/kg/hr (n = 18) dosage. Fibrinogen values on the dotted line were determined by the sodium sulfite method, and values on the solid line were determined by the Clauss clotting rate assay. Fibrinogen was sampled after 2, 4, and 6 hr of infusion and 24 hr after infusion.

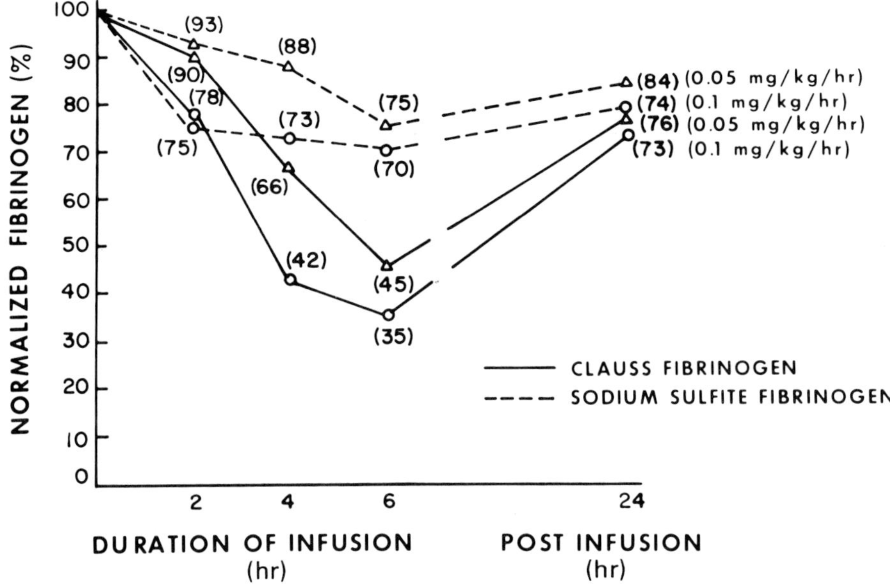

Figure 4   Comparative plotting of mean decreases of normalized α_2-antiplasmin values for rt-PA-treated patients receiving 0.1-mg/kg/hr (solid line) and 0.05-mg/kg/hr (dotted line) dosages. α_2-antiplasmin was sampled after 2, 4, and 6 hr of infusion and 24 hr after infusion. Differences observed after 2 hr of infusion are significant ($p < 0.05$).

mg/kg/hr dosage, plasminogen levels decreased an average of 50%. Again, in none was there complete depletion of circulating plasminogen.

Levels of circulating fibrin(ogen) degradation products ranged from 80 to 2560 µg/ml (average concentration 640 µg/ml). These levels did not differ in the groups receiving 0.1 to 0.05 mg/kg/hr. Absolute values for TT, PT, and APTT were not significantly prolonged in any patient.

V. COMPLICATIONS

During the infusions, small hematomas developed at the catheter entry site in eight of 55 patients (15%). These were all controlled by manual compression, and hemostasis was achieved immediately on withdrawal of the infusion catheter. Transfusions were not required, and no significant changes in hematocrits were observed. No allergic or other adverse reactions occurred.

In three patients, large hematomas formed concurrent with rt-PA infusion. In one of these patients receiving 0.05 mg/kg/hr of rt-PA, a calf hematoma developed due to the disruption of the distal anastomosis after the thrombus in a saphenous-vein femorotibial bypass graft was successfully lysed. The hematoma was evacuated at the time of surgical revision of the distal anastomosis. This led to no further clinical problems. A second patient developed a large groin hematoma requiring transfusion and one unit of packed red blood cells. This patient had heparin-associated white clot syndrome and was thrombocytopenic during the t-PA infusion. Hemostasis was controlled with local pressure. The third patient also had a distal graft anastomosis leak that required transfusion of blood products and surgical repair.

One patient while receiving intravenous heparin died from an intracranial hemorrhage 48 hr after the treatment with rt-PA (0.1 mg/kg/hr).

VI. DISCUSSION

Application of thrombolysis to peripheral artery and bypass graft occlusions began in the early 1970s when various doses of streptokinase were applied directly to the clot (1). Initially, the results were discouraging due to the long duration of infusion and resultant systemic "lytic state" (despite low-dose infusion technique) and excessive complication rates (3,4,7,8,19–22). Refinement of the technique and the development of rt-PA have now yielded encouraging results.

Urokinase, another effective thrombolytic agent, has not been used as commonly due to its increased cost. Urokinase possesses several advantages over streptokinase. The first and paramount advantage is that it is more gentle on the constituents of the fibrinolytic system, producing smaller decrements in circulating fibrinogen, and thereby leaving the patient less predisposed to bleeding complications. In addition, urokinase is rarely antigenic; it is not likely to cause the unpleasant side effects that are common with streptokinase. In general, the treatment duration with urokinase is shorter, thus decreasing to some degree the issue of cost (6).

Recombinant human tissue-type plasminogen activator appears to possess all the beneficial effects of urokinase and seems to be a more potent and a somewhat more fibrin-specific thrombolytic agent. In addition, rt-PA produces more rapid effect, allowing shorter durations of infusion and safer thrombus lysis by producing less alteration of the fibrinolytic and hemostatic blood constituents than do streptokinase and conventional dosages of urokinase (8,14). Initial studies with rt-PA have indicated that successful thrombolysis in a very rapid and safe fashion can be achieved in animal models and patients with acute coronary artery occlusion (12,13,17,23–28). Our initial studies (29–31) with rt-PA in peripheral artery and bypass graft occlusions demonstrate nearly uniform thrombolysis and significant fibrinogen-sparing when compared to a similar group of patients treated with streptokinase (8,29) (Figure 5). Although a comparison based on data from a retrospective control group treated with streptokinase is problematic, the patient populations, endpoints of treatment, and laboratory methodology were very comparable. Finally, the extent to which a more favorable laboratory profile will be accompanied by reduced incidence of bleeding remains to be established, but it is likely that the risk-benefit ratio will be improved.

Only four of 55 attempts at thrombolysis were unsuccessful, and in these patients inability to selectively catheterize the thrombosed femoropopliteal bypass graft seemed to preclude thrombolysis in two of the four. These data tend to support the intraarterial selective method of rt-PA infusion with the catheter embedded into the thrombus, although an intravenous infusion method study has not been systematically compared to the former method. In

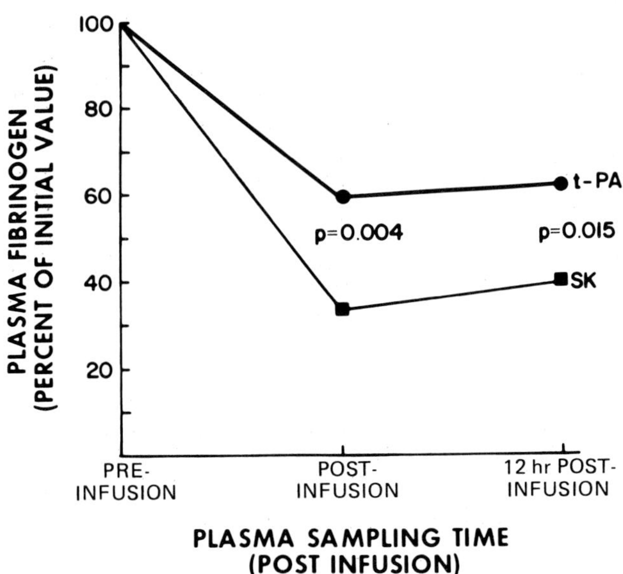

Figure 5   Mean fibrinogen depletion immediately and 12 hr after t-PA and streptokinase (SK) infusion.

the remaining two attempts, myointimal hyperplasia and atherosclerosis produced the occlusion or subtotal stenosis.

Time required for complete thrombus lysis with rt-PA varied from 1 to 8 hr, with a mean infusion time of 4.1 hr. In contrast, infusion durations in a similar group of patients who were treated with SK varied from 12 to 120 hr, with a mean infusion time of 51.3 hr (3). The ability to achieve thrombolysis did not appear to be affected by the thrombus age in the rt-PA-treated groups. All thrombi were less than 30 days in age (mean 7.5 days) clinically. Perhaps differences in rate or completeness of thrombus lysis may occur if rt-PA is applied clinically to "older" thrombi.

The decreases in plasma fibrinogen, plasminogen, and α_2-antiplasmin levels that occurred in our patient group indicate that a systemic lytic state can occur and is associated with varying degrees of fibrinogenolysis. In general, the pharmacodynamic effects of rt-PA on the systemic constituents of the fibrinolytic system are dependent on several factors. The initial concentration of α_2-antiplasmin and the participation of α_2-macroglobulin as an inhibitor and neutralizer of plasmin are important factors. Under circumstances in which the rapid inhibitor α_2-antiplasmin is depleted, a systemic lytic state is prevented until the slower inhibitor of plasmin, α_2-macroglobulin, is depleted. Previous studies (32) indicate that depletion of α_2-macroglobulin would predispose to a systemic lytic state as a result of plasmin elaboration in the circulation.

These pharmacodynamic effects are dependent not only on the concentration of these constituents but also on the duration of infusion and dosage administered. Tiefenbrunn et al. (32) and Verstraete et al. (33) have shown that as the duration of infusion increases, systemic lytic activity increases and fibrinogenolysis results. In most patients in our study, the size of the thrombus was much larger than in coronary artery infusions, and the duration of infusions was significantly longer. It is likely that longer infusion times can sufficiently deplete inhibitors of plasmin and result in systemic fibrinogen degradation. For example, a plasma concentration of rt-PA of 10 nM prevailing over 1-hr infusion would not yield significant systemic fibrinogenolysis. If this same concentration is maintained throughout a 6- or 8-hr infusion, one can predict that this will result in a more marked production of fibrinogenolysis (32).

Of additional importance, blood specimens must be protected from the in vitro artifact, which may account for the interstudy variation in the extent of fibrinogenolysis that has been seen in reported trials, despite similar rt-PA dosage regimens.

Attention to sample handling is important to prevent in vitro breakdown of fibrinogen. We took particular care to measure these proteins within 1 hr of obtaining the plasma, and the samples were supplemented with aprotinin and/or PPACK to prevent in vitro production of plasmin, which would have caused artifactual changes in the levels of the measured constituent.

Another possible explanation for discrepancies in fibrinogen levels is related to the methodology of fibrinogen determination. Many of the fibrinogen measurements in the coronary thrombolysis trials have been based on sodium sulfite or phosphate precipitation procedure. This method generally yields a higher level of fibrinogen as it is less sensitive to the effects of early degradation products. In an acute myocardial infarction study done by Verstraete et al. (13), a degree of fibrinogen breakdown similar to that in our patients was found when fibrinogen was measured by the clotting rate assay. A smaller decrease in fibrinogen concentration was seen when measured by the sodium sulfite method. The same observation has held in our patients when comparing the two modalities of fibrinogen determination (Figure 4).

Major bleeding complications occurred in three patients (5%) of 55 rt-PA treated patients. This complication rate is substantially lower than in most other studies using streptokinase or urokinase (2,6–8,21). Catheter-associated bleeding complications in the form of minor hematomas were few and easily controllable. In contrast, streptokinase-treated patients demonstrated gross derangements in hemostasis, causing much more difficulty in controlling catheter-associated bleeding problems.

More than one-half of the patients successfully treated with rt-PA required surgical intervention to repair or replace arteries or bypass grafts. The decision to perform surgical repair was based on anatomical considerations and not on the failure of anticoagulation. Arterial and bypass graft thrombolysis must be done in conjunction with a good vascular surgical team approach to allow repair or replacement of existing grafts or, on occasion, to allow rapid intervention in urgent situations such as graft anastomosis disruption. Early surgical intervention following rt-PA infusion was safe in our experience. Perhaps balloon angioplasty will be a more frequent alternative in our future patients, since the majority of these lesions surgically repaired were focal, and probably some were amenable to balloon angioplasty. Anticoagulation was used to prevent thrombosis in areas of tight stenosis until repair could be accomplished and also in patients with distal emboli or thrombosis to allow healing of the endothelium and prevent further embolization. rt-PA and heparin were not used concurrently in our study, and heparin probably is not required to prevent pericatheter thrombus formation. In fact, it will likely only contribute to an increase risk of bleeding.

The applicability of thrombolysis with rt-PA in the treatment of peripheral artery and bypass graft thrombosis remains to be definitively established. Thrombolysis may be preferable to surgical treatment in some patients, including individuals with arterial emboli (Figure 6) or thrombi, especially in

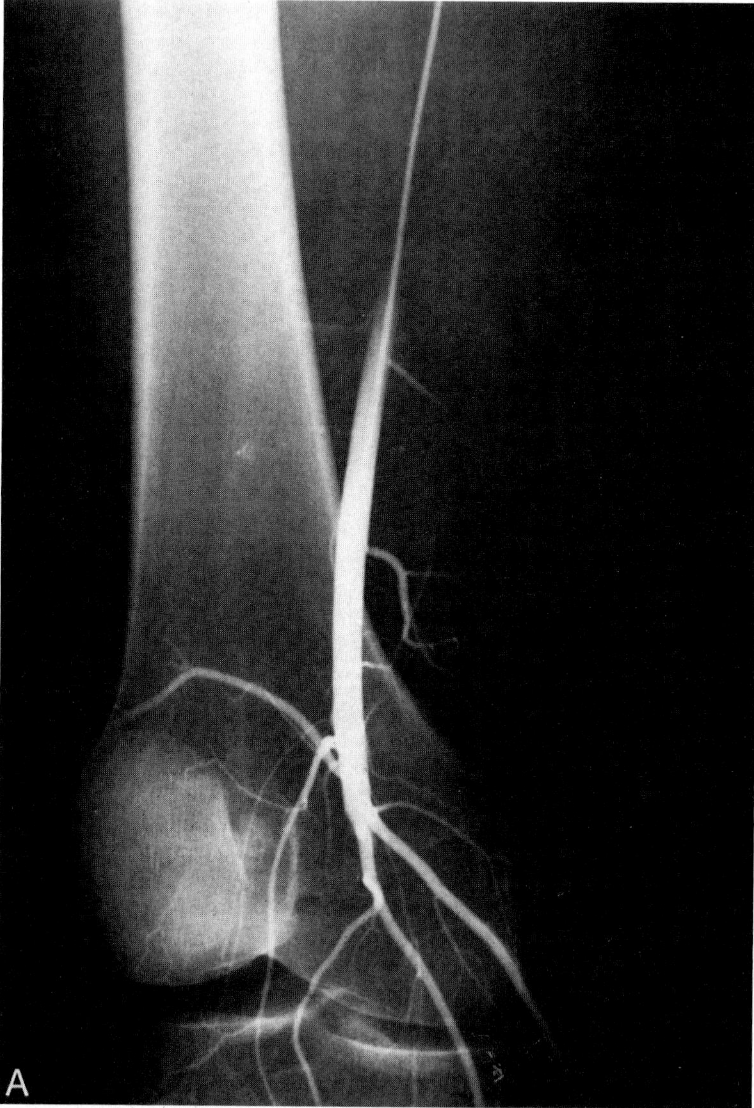

Figure 6   (A, B) Right femoral arteriogram demonstrates embolic occlusion of the popliteal artery with reconstitution of tibial vessels in a 28-year-old man with short-distance claudication of 3 weeks' duration. (C) Following 8 hr of rt-PA infusion, there has been extensive thrombus lysis within the popliteal and tibial arteries and re-establishment of flow into the foot (not shown). A small, nonoccluding thrombus remains in the popliteal artery.

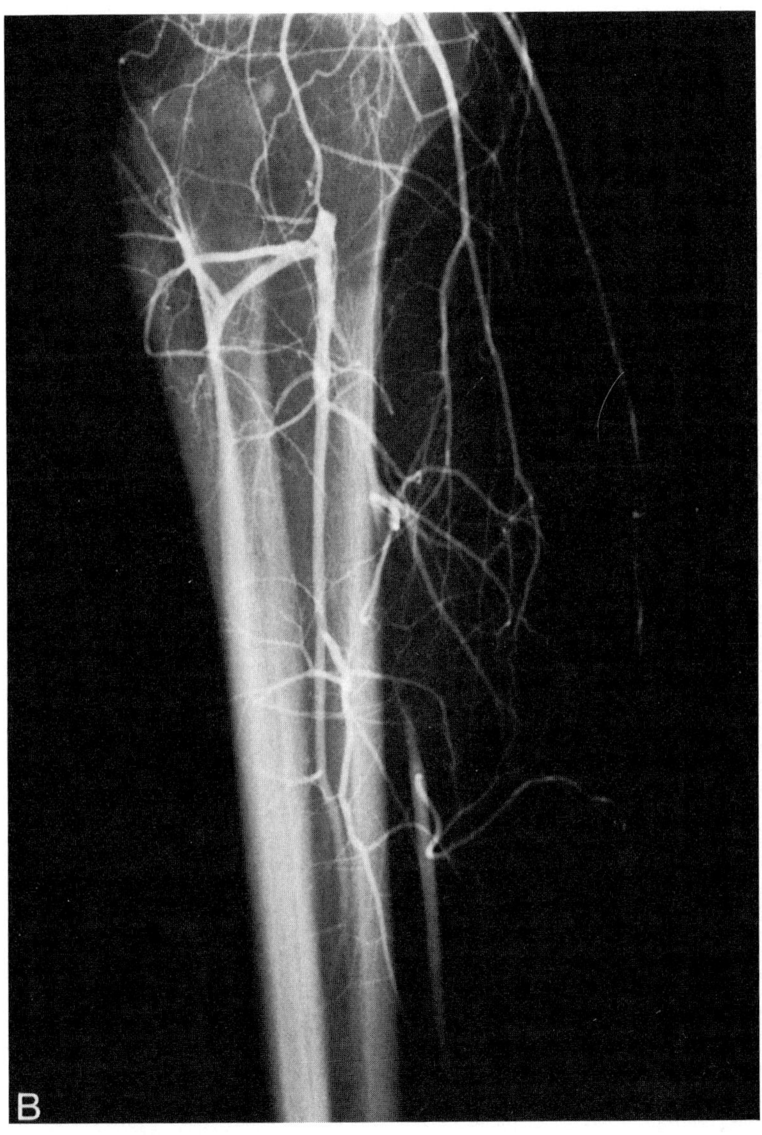
B

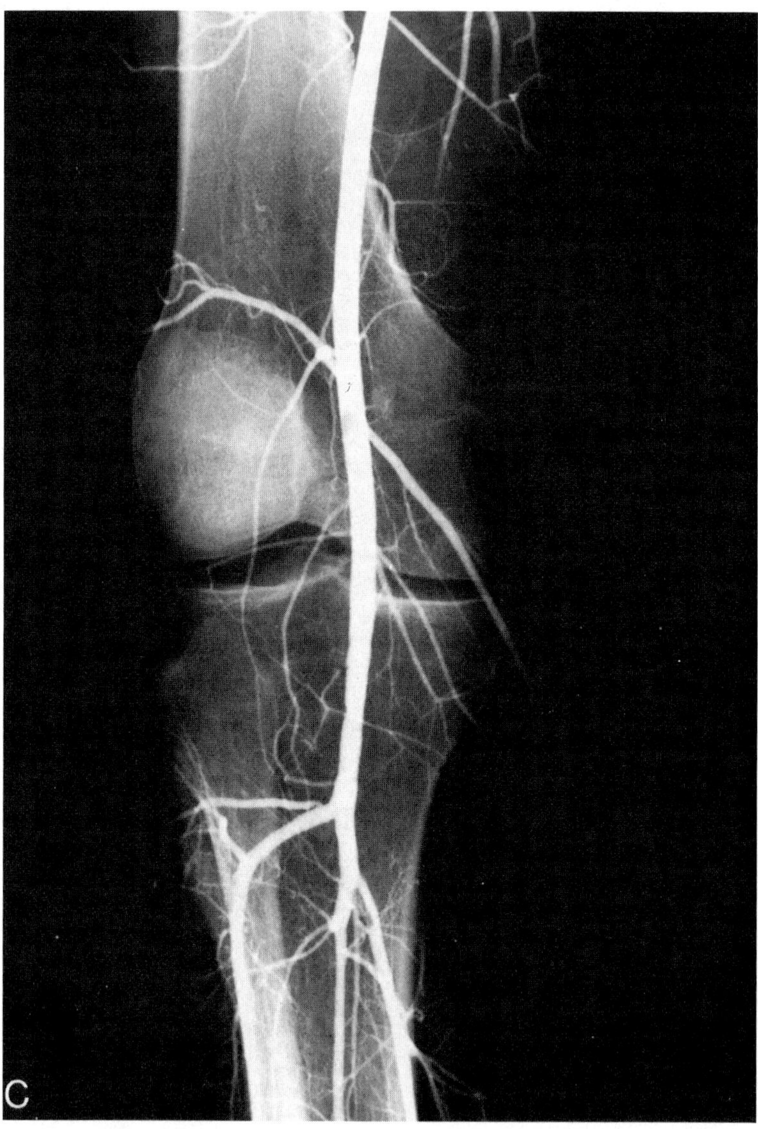

Figure 10.6 (Continued)

those with these conditions in small arteries partially or totally inaccessible to balloon catheter thrombectomy or embolectomy (Figure 7). A second group of patients in whom thrombolysis may be advantageous are those with thrombosed saphenous-vein bypass grafts. Preservation of the vein bypass may be better achieved with rt-PA so that endothelial damage that can result from balloon catheter thrombectomy can be avoided (Figure 8). A third situation where rt-PA may be advantageous is when the ischemic limb is determined angiographically inoperable. In this setting, rt-PA may reestablish flow in arteries adequate to accept bypass grafts or provide other alternatives. In addition, we have been successful in lowering the level of amputation in several patients by lysing thrombi in small arteries (e.g., distal branches of the profunda femoris). Other situations may be appropriate for rt-PA treatment, although adequate data are not available to establish definitive indications.

Further studies should help delineate the best method of administration of rt-PA necessary to produce thrombolysis and yet protect the patient from systemic fibrinogenolysis. It is also clear that clot sensitivity of rt-PA is not absolute, but is dependent on the extent to which fibrinolytic constituents such as α_2-antiplasmin and α_2-macroglobulin are consumed, and probably also to the duration of exogenous administration of rt-PA.

VI. CONCLUSION

In summary, the results of our study suggest that rt-PA is both safe and effective as a thrombolytic agent in the treatment of peripheral artery and bypass graft thrombosis. rt-PA offers theoretical advantages over conventional lytic agents and appears to be a very useful agent from a practical standpoint as well. Refinements in dose and laboratory technique for monitoring of patients receiving rt-PA have occurred and will likely undergo further fine-tuning.

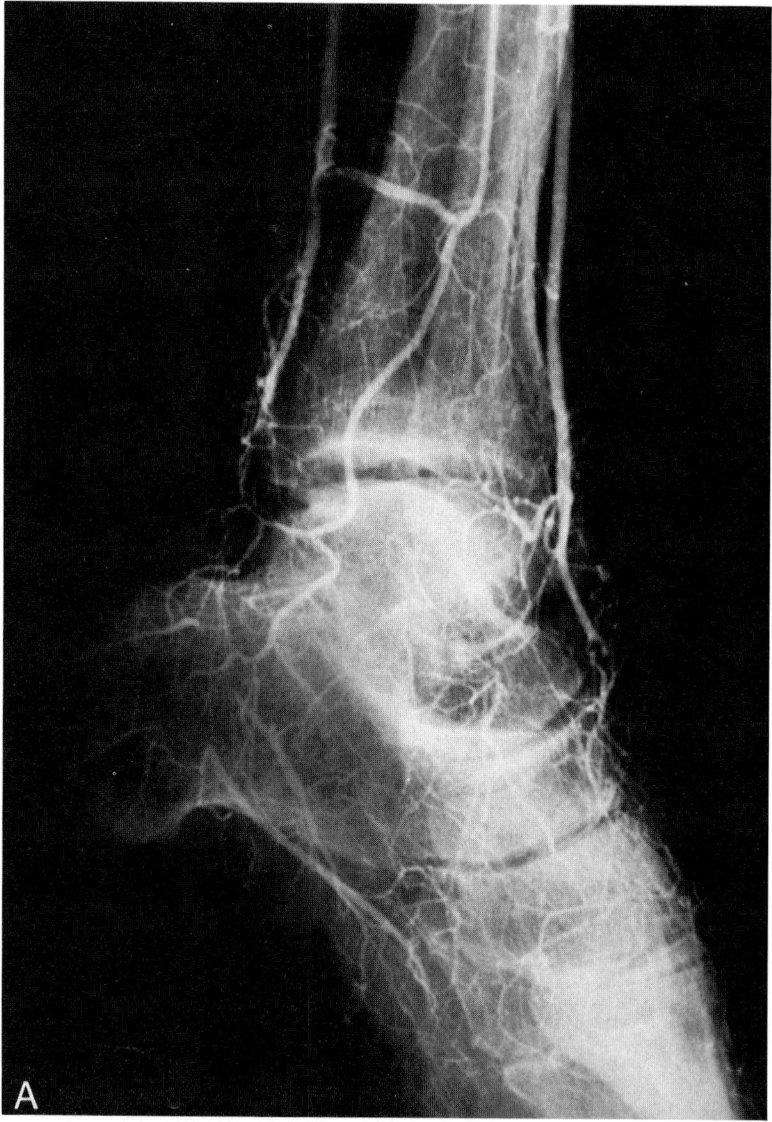

Figure 7   (A) Arteriogram of the right foot demonstrates occlusion of the anterior tibial and posterior tibial arteries in a 58-year-old man with a 2-week history of ischemic rest pain following embolization during aortic aneurysm resection. (B) Digital subtraction angiogram following rt-PA infusion in the posterior tibial artery demonstrates complete thrombus lysis in the posterior tibial artery. More distal films (not shown) demonstrated opacification of the plantar arch vessels to the level of metatarsal heads.

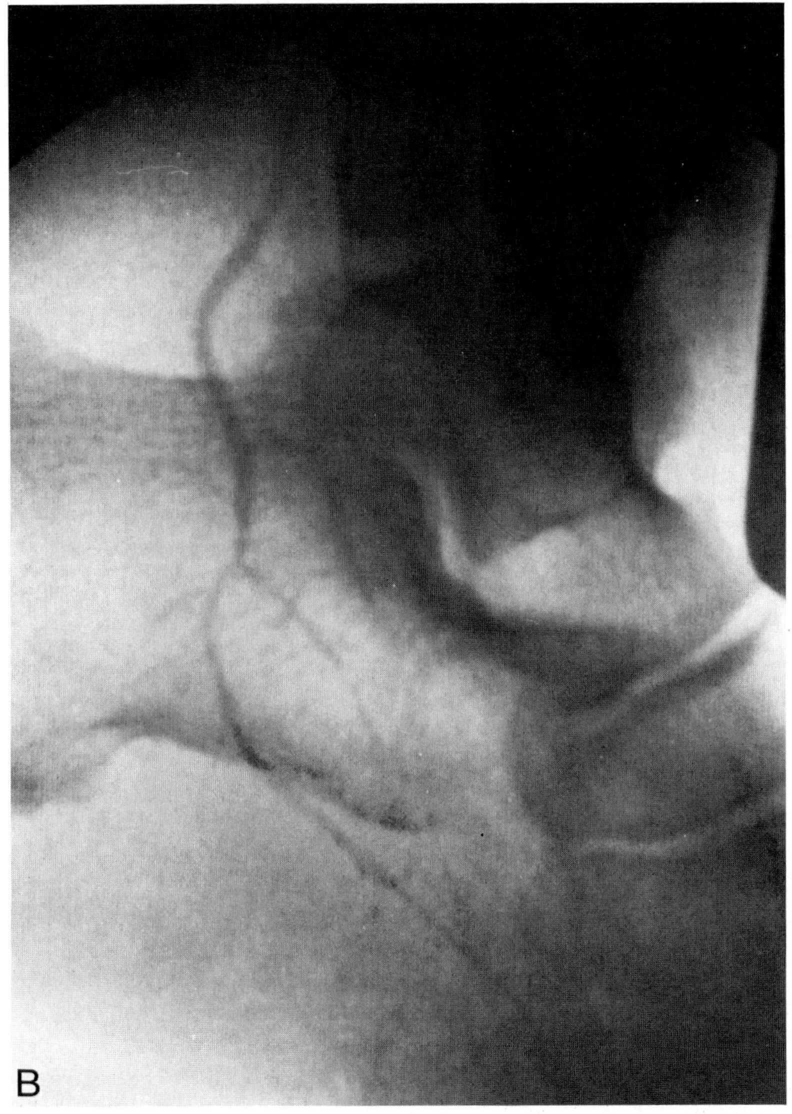

B

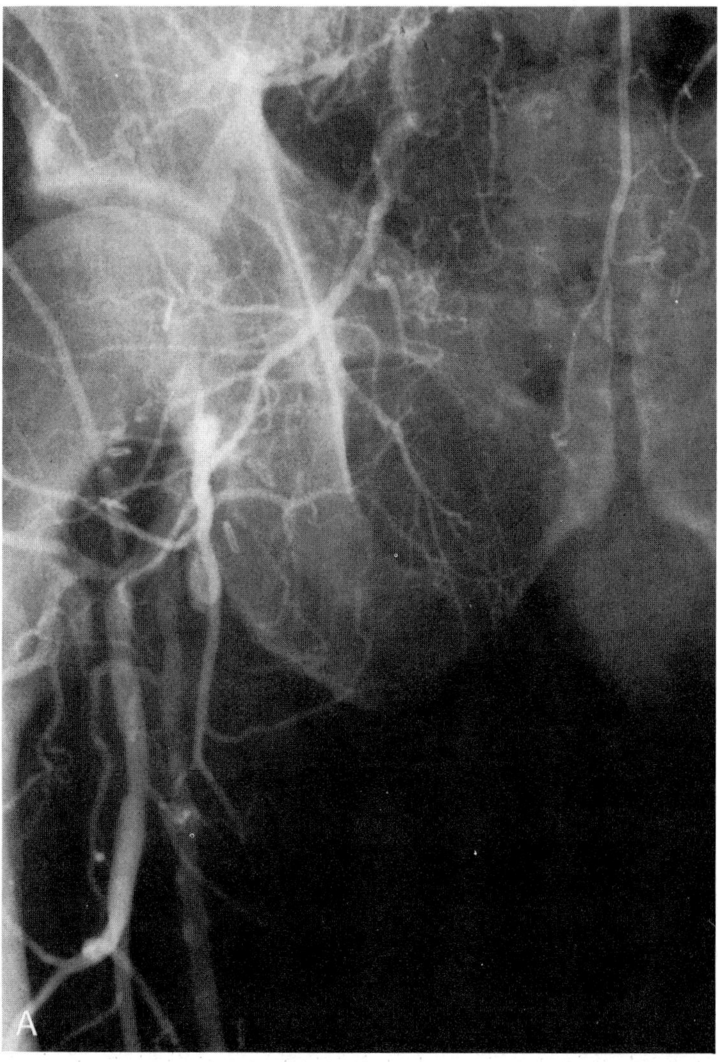

Figure 8   Right femoral arteriogram demonstrates occlusion of the right femoral popliteal bypass graft at its origin and occlusion of the superficial femoral artery in Hunter's canal, with only a few small collaterals identified about the knee and no opacification of the tibial vessels. The patient is a 65-year-old man with ischemic rest pain of 2 days' duration. Following 6 hr of rt-PA infusion, there has been complete thrombus lysis within the graft, popliteal, anterior, and posterior tibial arteries, with flow being reestablished into the foot. A postsurgical defect is identified at the distal anastomosis of the bypass graft.

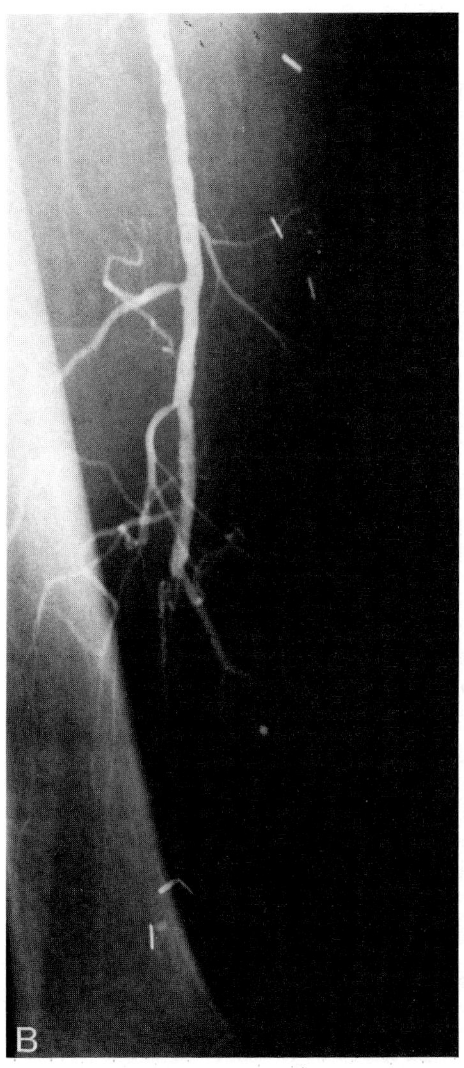

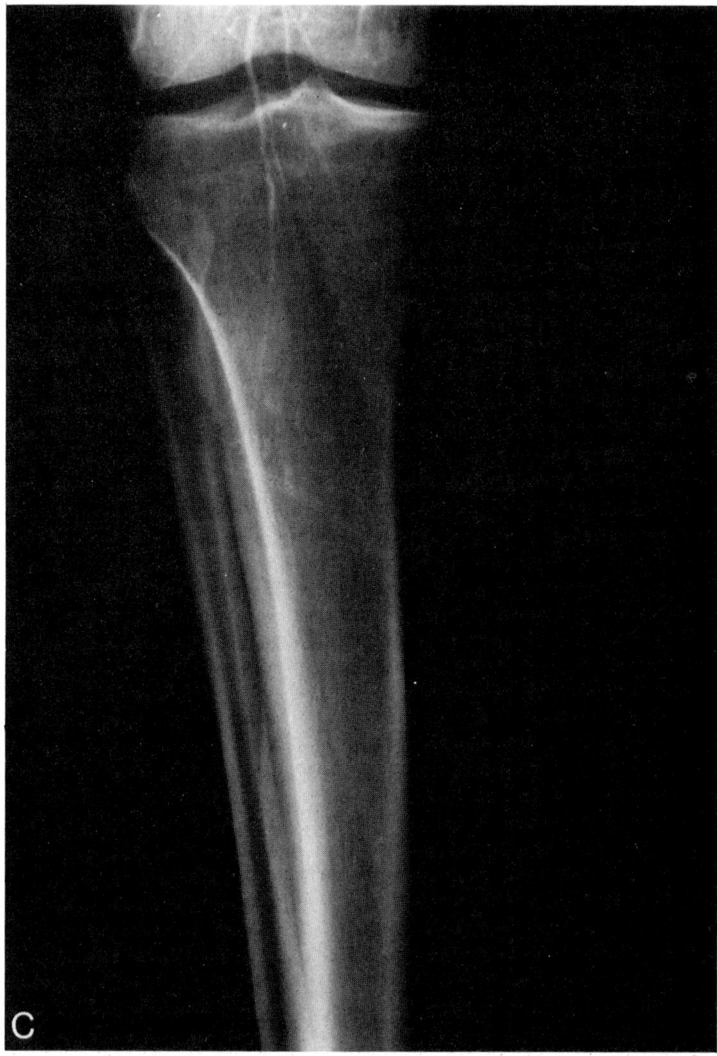

Figure 10.8 (Continued)

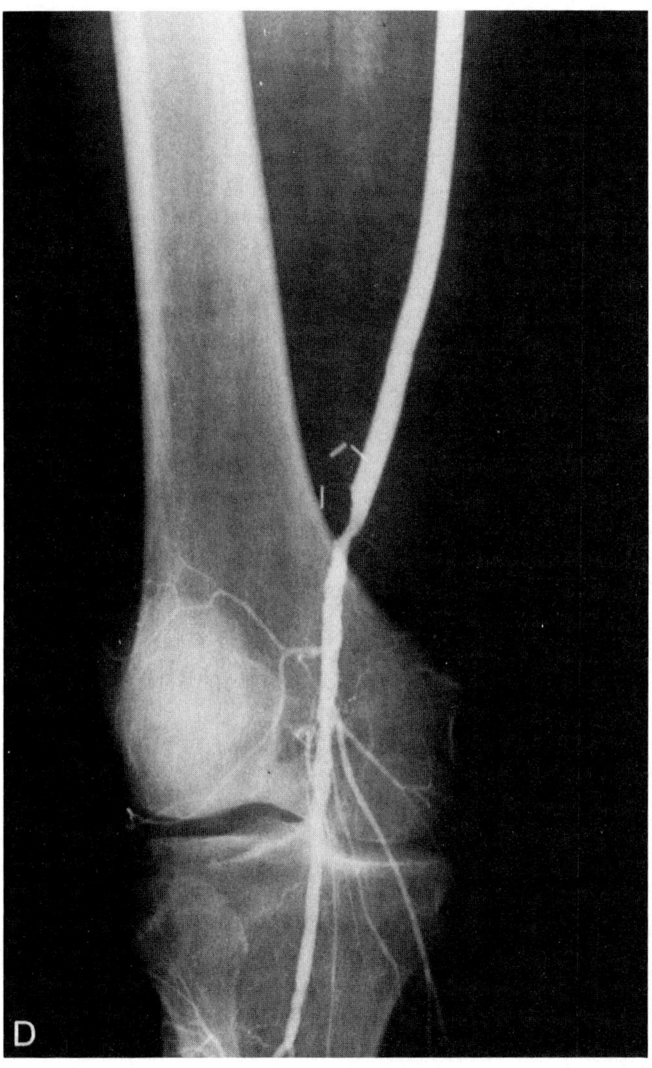

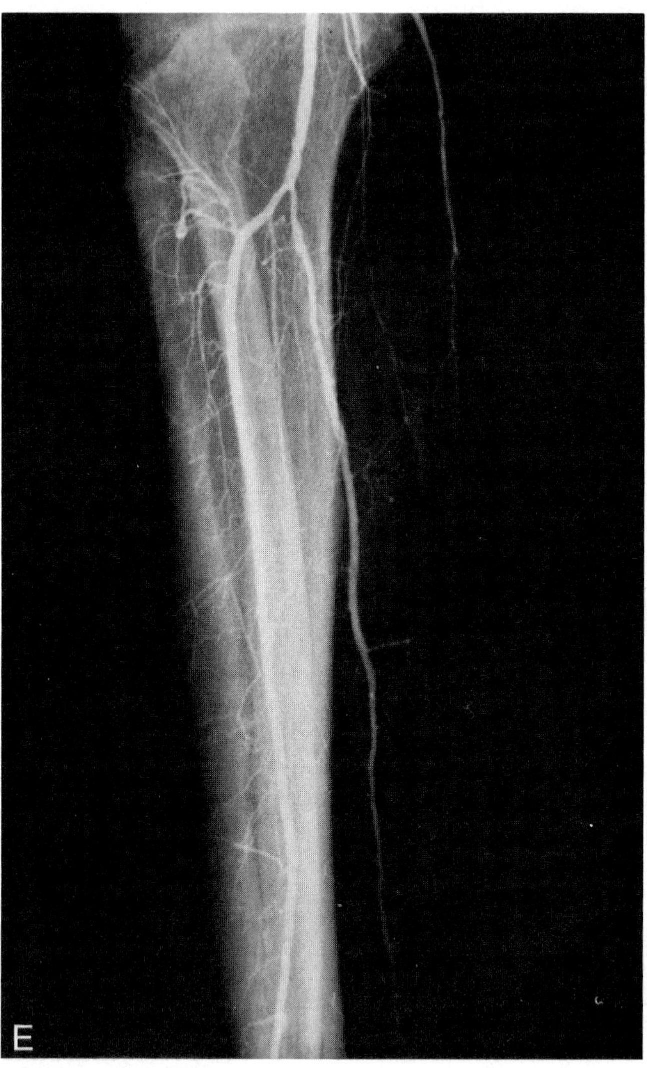

Figure 10.8 (Continued)

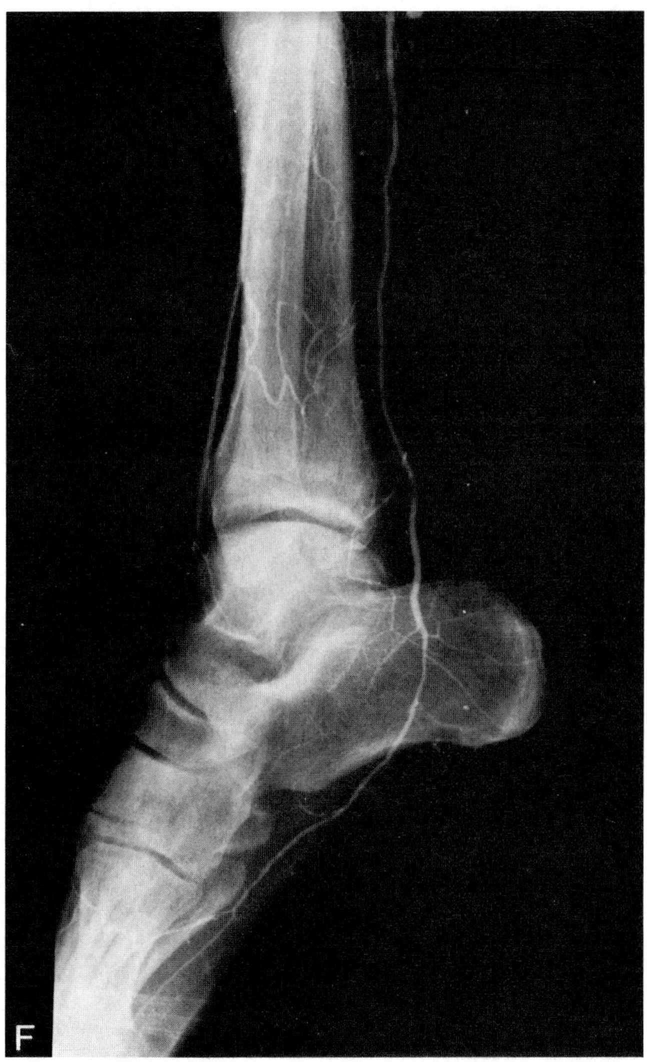
F

REFERENCES

1. Dotter CT, Rösh J, Seaman AJ: Selective clot lysis with low dose streptokinase. Radiology 111:31–37, 1974.
2. Katzen BTA, van Breda A: Low dose streptokinase in the treatment of arterial occlusions. AJR 136:1171–1178, 1981.
3. Graor RA, Risius B, Denny KM, Young JR, Beven EG, Hertzer NR, Ruschhaupt III WF, O'Hara PJ, Geisinger MA, Zelch MG: Local thrombolysis in the treatment of thrombosed arteries, bypass grafts, and arteriovenous fistulas. J Vasc Surg 2:406–414, 1985.
4. Hargrove WC, Berkowitz HD, Freiman DB, McLean G, Ring EJ, Roberts B: Recanalization of totally occluded femoropopliteal vein grafts with low dose streptokinase infusion. Surgery 92:890–895, 1982.
5. Risius B, Zelch MG, Graor RA, Geisinger MA, Smith JAM, Piraino DW: Catheter-directed low dose streptokinase infusion: A preliminary experience. Radiology 150:349–355, 1984.
6. McNamara TO, Fischer JR: Thrombolysis of peripheral arterial and graft occlusions: Improved results using high-dose urokinase. AJR 144:769–775, 1985.
7. VanBreda A, Robison JC, Feldman L, et al: Local thrombolysis in the treatment of arterial graft occlusions. J Vasc Surg 1:103–112, 1984.
8. Graor RA, Risius B, Young JR, Geisinger MA, Zelch MG, Smith JAM, Ruschhaupt WF: Low dose streptokinase for selective thrombus lysis: Systemic effects and complications. Radiology 152:35–39, 1984.
9. Totty WG, Gilula LA, McClennan BL, Ahmed P, Sherman L: Low-dose intravascular fibrinolytic therapy. Radiology 143:59–69, 1982.
10. Van de Werf F, Ludbrook PA, Bergmann SR, Tiefenbrunn AJ, Fox KAA, deGeest H, Verstraete M, Collen D, Sobel BE: Coronary thrombolysis with tissue-type plasminogen activator in patients with evolving myocardial infarction. N Engl J Med 310:609, 1984.
11. Collen D, Topol EJ, Tiefenbrunn AJ, Gold HK, Weisfeldt ML, Sobel BE, Leinbach RC, Brinker JA, Ludbrook PA, Yasuda I, Bulkley BH, Robison AK, Hutter AM, Bell WR, Spadara JJ, Khaw BA, Grossbard EB: Coronary thrombolysis with recombinant human tissue-type plasminogen activator: A prospective, randomized, placebo-controlled trial. Circulation 70:1012, 1984.
12. The TIMI study group: The thrombolysis in myocardial infarction (TIMI) trial: phase I findings. N Engl J Med 312:932, 1985.
13. Verstraete M, Bernard R, Bory M, Brower RW, Collen D, DeBone DP, Erbel R, Huhmann W, Lennane RJ, Lubsen J, Mathey D, Meyer J, Michels HR, Rutsch W, Schartl M, Schmidt W, Uebis R, von Essen R: Randomized trial of intravenous recombinant tissue-type plasminogen activator versus intravenous streptokinase in acute myocardial infarction. Lancet 2:842, 1985.
14. Tiefenbrunn A, Sobel BE: Tissue-type plasminogen activator (t-PA): An agent with promise for selective thrombolysis. Int J Cardiol 7:82, 1985.

15. Sobel BE, Gross RW, Robison AK: Thrombolysis, clot selectivity, and kinetics. Circulation 70:160, 1984.

16. Fox KAA, Robison AK, Knabb RM, Rosamond TL, Sobel BE, Bergmann SR: Prevention of coronary thrombosis with subthrombolytic doses of tissue-type plasminogen activator. Circulation 72:1346, 1985.

17. Collen D, Bounameaux H, DeCock F, Lijnen HR, Verstraete M: Analysis of coagulation and fibrinolysis during intravenous infusion of recombinant human tissue-type plasminogen activator in patients with acute myocardial infarction. Circulation 73:511, 1986.

18. Topol EJ, Bell WR, Weisfeldt ML: Coronary thrombolysis with recombinant tissue-type plasminogen activator. A hematologic and pharmacologic study. Ann Intern Med 103:837, 1985.

19. Becker GJ, Rabe FE, Richmond BD, et al: Low-dose fibrinolytic therapy. Radiology 148:663–670, 1983.

20. Wolfson RH, Kumpe DA, Rutherford RB: Role of intraarterial streptokinase in treatment of arterial thromboembolism. Arch Surg 119:697–702, 1984.

21. Becker GJ, Rabe FE, Richmond BD, Holden RW, Yune HY, Dilley RS, Bong NU, Glover JL, Klatte EC: Low-dose fibrinolytic therapy: Results and new concepts. Radiology 148:663–670, 1983.

22. Persson AV, Robichaux WT, Jaxheimer EC, DiPronio EM: Burst therapy: A method of administering fibrinolytic agents. Am J Surg 147:531–536, 1984.

23. Tiefenbrunn AJ, Robison AK, Kurnik PB, Ludbrook PA, Sobel BE: Clinical pharmacology in patients with evolving myocardial infarction of tissue-type plasminogen activator produced by recombinant DNA technology. Circulation 71:110, 1985.

24. Van de Werf F, Bergmann SR, Fox KAA, deGeest H, Hoyng CF, Sobel BE, Collen D: Coronary thrombolysis with intravenously administered human tissue-type plasminogen activator produced by recombinant DNA technology. Circulation 69:605–610, 1984.

25. Gold HK, Fallon JT, Yasuda T, Leinbach RC, Khaw BA, Newell JB, Guerrero JL, Vislosky FM, Hoyng CF, Grossbard E, Collen D: Coronary thrombolysis with recombinant human tissue-type plasminogen activator. Circulation 70:700–707, 1984.

26. Collen D, Topol EJ, Tiefenbrunn AJ, Gold HK, Weisfeldt ML, Sobel BE, Leinbach RC, Brinker JA, Ludbrook PA, Yasuda I, Bulkley BH, Robison AK, Hutter AM, Bell WB, Spadaro JJ, Khaw BA, Grossbard EB: Coronary thrombolysis with recombinant human tissue-type plasminogen activator: A prospective, randomized, placebo-controlled trial. Circulation 70:1012–1017, 1984.

27. Van de Werf F, Ludbrook PA, Bergmann SR, Tiefenbrunn AJ, Fox KAA, deGeest H, Verstraete M, Collen D, Sobel BE: Coronary thrombolysis with tissue-type plasminogen activator in patients with evolving myocardial infarction. N Engl J Med 310:609, 1984.

28. Verstraete M, Bounameaux H, DeCock F, Van de Werf F, Collen D: Phar-

macokinetics and systemic fibrinogenolytic effects of recombinant human tissue-type plasminogen activator in man. J Pharmacol Exp Ther 235:506–512, 1985.

29. Graor RA, Risius B, Young JR, et al: Peripheral artery and bypass graft thrombolysis with recombinant human tissue-type plasminogen activator. J Vasc Surg 3:115–124, 1986.

30. Risius B, Graor RA, Geisinger MA, et al: Recombinant tissue-type plasminogen activator for thrombolysis in peripheral arteries and bypass grafts. Radiology 160:183–188, 1986.

31. Graor RA, Risius B, Lucas FV, et al: Thrombolysis with recombinant human tissue-type plasminogen activator in patients with peripheral artery and bypass graft occlusions. Circulation 74(suppl I):1, 1986.

32. Tiefenbrunn AJ, Graor RA, Robison AK, Lucas FV, Hotchkiss A, Sobel BE: Pharmacodynamics of tissue-type plasminogen activator characterized by computer-assisted simulation. Circulation 73:1291–1299, 1986.

33. Verstraete M, Bory M, Collen D, et al: Randomized trial of intravenous recombinant tissue-type plasminogen activator versus intravenous streptokinase in acute myocardial infarction. Lancet 2:842–847, 1985.

THE EUROPEAN AND JAPANESE EXPERIENCE

11

The European Experience with Recombinant Tissue-Type Plasminogen Activator in Acute Myocardial Infarction

Marc Verstraete
University of Leuven
Leuven, Belgium

When recombinant tissue-type plasminogen activator (rt-PA) became available for clinical investigation in Europe, two randomized multicenter trials in patients with acute first myocardial infarction were launched simultaneously by the European Cooperative Study Group for Recombinant Tissue-Type Plasminogen Activator (members are listed in the Appendix). The relative effectiveness in terms of angiographically proven coronary patency of intravenously administered rt-PA was compared with that of placebo in six European centers and with that of streptokinase in seven other centers. Further aims were to compare the safety of the different drug regimens and to assess their effect on components of the coagulation and fibrinolytic system.

I. PATIENT SELECTION AND EXPERIMENTAL PROTOCOL

The criteria used for patient selection were the same in the two trials (1,2). In brief, patients less than 70 years old hospitalized within 6 hr of onset of symptoms of a first infarction were eligible for participation, provided that severe chest pain lasted for at least 30 min and that the electrocardiogram showed an acute injury pattern (at least a 2-mm ST-segment elevation 60 ms after J-point, in two or more standard frontal leads, or 3 mm in two or more precordial leads). Cardiogenic shock was an exclusion criterion as were the usual contraindications for the administration of thrombolytic drugs. After having obtained informed consent, the enrolling physician telephoned identification of an eligible patient to the Data Center. The Data Center then instructed the investigator as to which coded prepackaged vials, containing either rt-PA or the alternative substance, were to be administered. Allocation was at random and balanced per clinic.

On presentation to the emergency room, the patient received conventional therapy for acute myocardial infarction. Blood was drawn for enzyme and coagulation factor determination. A bolus intravenous injection of 5000 IU heparin was given to all patients and followed by intravenous infusion of either rt-PA (0.75 mg/kg body weight) or placebo over 90 min in the double-blind trial (1) or by the same dose of rt-PA or 1,500,000 IU streptokinase in the single-blind trial (2). The latter subgroup also received 0.5 g methyl prednisone and 0.5 g acetylsalicylic acid intravenously just prior to streptokinase, which was administered by infusion pump over 60 min. The shorter infusion period of streptokinase (60 min) compared with rt-PA (90 min) was chosen to be in line with the major clinical trials using a high-dose, brief-duration streptokinase regimen.

Selective coronary arteriography was performed between 75 and 90 min after the start of the infusion of the trial drug. Individual centers were free to choose between the Sones and Judkins techniques, and to decide which coronary vessel to inject first. At least two views were required of the right coronary artery and three of the left. Coronary angiography was recorded on 35-mm cinefilm, and this record, as evaluated by the independent Angiography Evaluation Group, represented the primary endpoint of the study. Once angiography had been performed, all subsequent diagnostic or therapeutic procedures were at the discretion of the individual centers. No antiarrhythmic drugs were given prophylactically, but they were used as required. Analgesics were given ad libitum. All medication used was recorded on the trial proforma. Treatment after coronary angiography was left to the discretion of the investigator.

II. ASSESSMENT OF CORONARY ANGIOGRAMS

Each cardiogram was read centrally by two assessors from a panel of experienced cardiologists and radiologists. The assessors knew the code number of the arteriogram, and whether or not the electrocardiogram at the time of entry showed ST elevation in leads V_2, V_3, and V_4. They were blinded to patient identity and treatment assignment.

Each assessor scored the arteriogram individually, segment by segment, and recorded the results of visual assessment on a standard proforma using a predetermined qualitative code: 0, normal vessel; 1, mild stenosis less than 50% of the vessel diameter; 2, moderate stenosis greater than 50% but less than 90%; 3, severe stenosis greater than 90%, but distal vessels fill completely, not through collaterals, within three cardiac cycles; 4, subtotal occlusion, distal vessel does not fill within three cardiac cycles; and 5, total occlusion with or without collateral filling. Collateral filling and left or right dominance were recorded, and the technical quality of the angiogram assessed on a 10-point scale. In some angiograms, a vessel filled poorly on the first injection of contrast, but subsequent injections showed better filling, either because of contrast-induced vasodilation or because thrombus was displaced. These angiograms were scored on the basis of the *first* technically adequate injection. Each assessor decided independently whether the presumed infarct vessel was patent, nonpatent, or impossible to assess. Patency was defined as all the vessels in the infarct-related area having scores of 3 or less with no "missing vessels." The infarct-related vessel was considered to be nonpatent if any of the vessels in the infarct-related area was seen as a totally occluded stump (code 5) or a subtotally occluded vessel with poor distal filling (code 4). At the end of the session, the two assessors compared their reports and reviewed any arteriograms that were discrepant.

III. ANALYSIS OF BLOOD SAMPLES FOR COAGULATION AND FIBRINOLYTIC ASSAYS

In addition to enzyme and other analyses performed in each medical center, blood samples were collected in these two studies for analysis in the Central Coagulation Laboratory. Fibrinogen was measured by means of a clotting rate assay (3) and a sodium sulfite precipitation method (4). Fibrin degradation products (5) and rt-PA-antigen (6) were also determined.

IV. COMPARISON OF THE STUDY GROUPS BEFORE TRIAL TREATMENT

The two groups in each trial were similar with respect to sex ratio, age, location of infarction, cardiovascular parameters, and the interval between the onset of pain and the initiation of infusion (3 hr). Also, the baseline serum enzyme levels were similar in the two treatment groups of each trial. Measurement of rt-PA levels and fibrinolytic activity in blood confirmed the correct allocation of treatment, and the clinicians reported that the full treatment dose was administered in all patients except one in the streptokinase group because shock developed and another in the placebo group because the ECG had normalized before the infusion was started. The final diagnosis of transmural infarction was confirmed by electrocardiographic evaluation and myocardial blood-enzyme elevation in 116 patients or by ECG in the remaining 12 of the 128 patients admitted to the double-blind, placebo-controlled trial. A transmural infarction was confirmed in the 128 patients of the second trial; in 97% this was based on a diagnostic ECG pattern together with a typical increase of blood-enzyme levels.

V. ANGIOGRAPHIC RESULTS

rt-PA Versus Placebo Trial

The angiographic outcome was not defined in five patients. In two of three patients assigned to placebo the angiograms were of poor quality, and in the third the attending physician decided not to complete the protocol because the ECG had normalized before the infusion would have been started. All documents for one patient treated with rt-PA were lost. For one patient assigned to rt-PA, fluoroscopy could not be performed because of equipment failure. The numbers of patients with assessable angiograms with patent or nonpatent infarct-related arteries in each center are shown in Table 1. Combining the results from all centers, the infarct-related arteries were classified as patent in 38 of 62 patients (61%) treated with rt-PA and in 13 of 62 patients (21%) of the placebo group who had an assessable coronary angiogram. This 40% difference in patency rate is significant ($p < 0.0001$; 95% confidence interval 24 to 55%). Of the 24 angiograms assessed as nonpatent (grades 4 or 5), eight had a subtotal occlusion (grade 4) in the rt-PA-treated patients. The corresponding figure for the placebo group is 7 (grade 4) on 49 nonpatent presumed infarct-related coronary arteries. The difference in patency rates between centers are not significant. In 29 of 73 patients in whom the infarct-related artery was still occluded at angiography, subsequent revascularization was attempted. In six of 24 patients initially treated with rt-PA, intracoronary streptokinase (five patients) or urokinase (one patient) was given; reperfusion was obtained in five of these. Similarly, intracoronary streptokinase was started following infusion of placebo in 15 of the 49 patients of this group; reperfusion was obtained in 12 patients. More patients were subjected to urgent percutaneous transluminal angioplasty in the placebo group (eight patients) than in the rt-PA-treated group (two patients). Except for two pa-

Table 1   Status of Presumed Infarct-Related Coronary Artery as Assessed by the Angiography Evaluation Group

	Placebo group	rt-PA group	Streptokinase group	rt-PA group
Assessed as patent (grades 0–3)	13 (21%)	38 (61%)	34 (55%)	43 (70%)
Assessed as nonpatent (grades 4–5)	49	24	28	18
subtotal occlusion (grade 4)	7	8	12	5
total occlusion (grade 5)	0	0	16	13
Not assessable	3[a]	2[b]	0	2[c]
Total	62	62	62	61/64

[a]In two patients the angiograms were of poor quality; in one patient the ECGs became normal before ECG should have started.
[b]All documents lost for one patient, fluoroscopy broken for another.
[c]Angiograms not performed for technical reasons in two patients.

tients, this mechanical treatment was associated with intracoronary infusion of streptokinase, and in these 10 patients reperfusion was achieved.

rt-PA Versus Streptokinase Trial

The numbers of patients with occluded or subtotally occluded infarct-related vessels and patients with patent vessels in each treatment group are shown in Table 1. There is a 15% group difference in favor of the rt-PA treatment (70% in the rt-PA-treated group and 55% in the streptokinase-treated group); the 95% confidence intervals of this difference range from +32 to −2% (p = 0.054).

VI. COMPLICATIONS DURING INFUSION UNTIL DISCHARGE

rt-PA Versus Placebo Trial

The infusion of rt-PA was well tolerated.

Major hemorrhagic complications were not encountered *during* infusion or cardiac catheterization, and there were no signs of central nervous system

Table 2   Events During Infusion Until Discharge

	Placebo group	rt-PA group	Streptokinase group	rt-PA group
Definite reinfarction	0	3	4	2
Signs of bleeding	5	11	34	17
Blood transfusion given	4	1	5	4

bleeding. In three patients treated with rt-PA, but in none of the control group, minor bleeding, mainly at arterial puncture sites, was noted during infusion of rt-PA and ceased when local pressure was applied (Table 2). None of the seven patients who developed a systolic blood pressure below 90 mm Hg had signs of bleeding.

There were few bleeding complications *after* rt-PA or placebo infusion, not requiring blood transfusion except in one patient on the third day after placebo infusion (Table 2). One rt-PA-treated patient received cimetidine for gastrointestinal bleeding, and one patient in the placebo group had nasal bleeding requiring tamponade. Other bleeding complications did not require special measures or were controlled by local pressure at the arterial puncture site. After infusion, chest pain without reinfarction was more common in the rt-PA-treated group; there were three patients treated with rt-PA who experienced a definite reinfarction during their hospital stay but none of the placebo patients did so.

rt-PA Versus Streptokinase Trial

Streptokinase infusion was also well tolerated. Minor hemorrhagic complications, mainly bleeding at puncture sites, were rare and did not occur more frequently during infusion in one of the two treatment groups. No blood transfusion had to be given during the brief period of infusion and heart catheterization. During the first 48 hr after transfer to the CCU, hematoma and prolonged bleeding at puncture sites were more frequently a problem in the streptokinase-treated patients, but blood transfusions were required equally rarely in the two treatment groups (Table 2). Retroperitoneal bleeding, cerebral hemorrhage, melena, and hematemesis did not occur in either treatment group. Only one patient had an allergic reaction; he had been treated with streptokinase. There was one transient ischemic episode during catheterization in an rt-PA-treated patient and a CVA in a streptokinase-treated patient who was discharged with a neurological deficit.

VII. COAGULATION AND FIBRINOLYTIC SYSTEM COMPONENTS

Intravenous infusion of 0.5 mg rt-PA/kg over 90 min resulted in steady-state rt-PA plasma antigen levels of 1.2 ± 0.6 µg/ml (n = 93) 60 min after start of infusion (7). These concentrations are about 1000 times higher than the baseline level in healthy subjects (8). The large standard variation confirms a considerable interindividual variability, as was already shown in pharmacokinetic studies in healthy volunteers (9) and in patients suffering from various pathological conditions (10). The variability in plasma rt-PA levels may reflect differences in the distribution volume of rt-PA but is more likely attributable to differences in turnover. Because rt-PA is eliminated almost exclusively by the liver (11,12), diminished hepatic blood flow may considerably affect the plasma half-life of rt-PA; it has been shown in rabbits that profound reduction of liver blood flow (to 12.5% of normal, a reduction much in excess of that seen with shock) results in a doubling of the plasma half-life of rt-PA (13).

The rt-PA activity assessed as plasma euglobulin fibrinolytic activity on fibrin plates correlated well with the circulating rt-PA antigen levels (r = 0.49; n = 0; $p < 0.001$), indicating that most of the rt-PA antigen circulates as free and active rt-PA.

Intravenous infusion of 0.75 mg rt-PA/kg over 90 min resulted in a decrease of the plasma fibrinogen level to $57 \pm 33\%$ of the baseline value at the end of the infusion (n = 89). Following intravenous infusion of 1,500,000 IU of streptokinase over 60 min, the fibrinogen level dropped to $11 \pm 18\%$ of the baseline level at the end of the infusion and to $7 \pm 10\%$ 30 min later (n = 56). In the placebo group, the fibrinogen breakdown was negligible. After 60 min of infusion, the fibrinogen level as measured with the clotting rate assay had dropped to below 1.0 g/L in nine out of 89 patients (10%) treated with rt-PA and in 50 out of 56 patients (89%) of the streptokinase-treated patients (Figure 1). Ninety minutes after the start of infusion, the corresponding figures were 24 out of 89 patients (27%) in the rt-PA group and 54 out of 57 (95%) in the streptokinase group. After 60 min of infusion, only one rt-PA-treated patient had a fibrinogen level below 0.5 g/L against 48 (86%) in the streptokinase group. The corresponding figures at 90 min were 10 out of 89 (11%) following rt-PA and 53 out of 57 (92%) following streptokinase. There was only a weak overall correlation between the fibrinogen breakdown and the plasma steady-state antigen levels of rt-PA (r = 0.21; n = 89; $0.1 > p >$

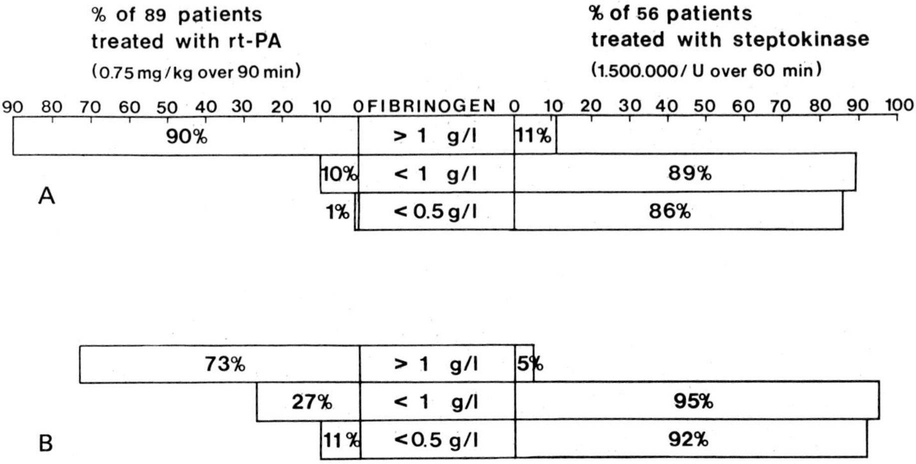

Figure 1   Value of fibrinogen in plasma (A) 60 and (B) 90 minutes after start of infusion.

0.05) (7). Some patients have a considerable decrease in circulating fibrinogen levels in the presence of relatively low concentrations of rt-PA. A possible explanation could be an ongoing low-grade, compensated, intravascular coagulation with presence of fibrin in the microcirculation. The extent of fibrinogen breakdown in rabbits was found to be directly proportional to the amount of injected fibrin (13). Extrapolation of observations in animals to patients with thromboembolic disease is hazardous, however. Fibrinogen breakdown in the rt-PA and streptokinase groups appeared to be less extensive when fibrinogen was assayed by sodium sulfite precipitation (4) which both rapidly assesses a coagulable fibrinogen and slowly assesses clottable fibrinogen degradation products such as fragments X and Y (7).

Fibrinogen-fibrin degradation products increased to 0.75 ± 0.54 mg/ml in the streptokinase group (n = 53), but only to 0.10 ± 0.13 mg/ml in the rt-PA group (n = 91) and to 0.02 ± 0.06 mg/ml in the placebo group (n = 37). These levels represent about 30% of the baseline fibrinogen level of 2.6 g/L in the streptokinase-treated patients and about 4% and 1% in the rt-PA (baseline fibrinogen 2.7 g/L) and the placebo (baseline fibrinogen 2.8 g/L) groups, respectively. The decrease of α_2-antiplasmin was extensive in the rt-PA- and streptokinase-treated groups but was significantly greater in the streptokinase-treated patients. Circulating plasminogen levels decreased twice as much in the streptokinase than in the rt-PA group (7).

On the basis of the kinetic parameters of the plasminogen activation by t-PA (14), the rate of plasmin formation may be represented by $V = (k_{cat}/K_m) \cdot [A] \cdot [P]$, where [A] equals plasma rt-PA concentration, [P] equals plasma concentration of plasminogen (2 μM), $k_{cat} = 0.1$ s^{-1}, and $K_m = 65$ μM. Consequently, at a plasma concentration of 1.5 μg of rt-PA per milliliter (0.02 μM), $v = 6.10^{-4}$ μM·s^{-1} or 0.2 μM·hr^{-1} (7). Thus, conversion of 10% of the circulating plasminogen and consumption of 20% of α_2-antiplasmin may be expected per hour under these conditions. This is in agreement with the results of a recent pharmacokinetic study in healthy volunteers in whom 40 or 60 mg of rt-PA administered over 90 min were compared, each dose being followed by a maintenance infusion of 30 mg of rt-PA over 6 hr; no further decrease of fibrinogen and plasminogen was observed between the beginning and end of the maintenance infusion (9).

All data discussed above refer to rt-PA as produced by Genentech on a small scale (G11021). A second preparation produced on a large scale (G11035) yielded, at comparable infusion rates, plasma rt-PA-antigen levels that were approximately 35% lower than with G11021 (p < 0.025) (15).

VIII. EARLY RETHROMBOSIS AFTER rt-PA-INDUCED RECANALIZATION

Rethrombosis is one of the major problems after coronary reperfusion with thrombolytic drugs. Clinically angiographic recognized reocclusion is most common in the days immediately following reperfusion, and estimates of the angiographic reocclusion rate during the first 10 days after thrombolytic treatment range from 9 to 46% (16,17). There has been concern that the short plasma half-life of rt-PA may increase the risk of early reocclusion (18,19). In a recent European trial, the risk of subsequent reocclusion was studied after patency of the infarct-related artery was obtained following an intravenous infusion of rt-PA (40 mg over 90 min) (20). A coronary angiogram was obtained after the first rt-PA infusion in 119 patients; the local cardiologists considered the infarct-related artery to be occluded in 33 and patent in the remaining 86 patients (72%) of this trial. The latter 86 patients received further heparin and were randomized to either an additional rt-PT infusion (30 mg over 6 hr) (n = 42) or placebo (n = 40). On central analysis of the second coronary angiogram, made 6 to 24 hr later, the reocclusion was 8%, without difference between the two treatment groups. With such an unexpected low incidence of early reocclusion, it was less surprising that no advantage of a second dose of rt-PA could be demonstrated with respect to further reduction of the reocclusion rate. The results of quantitative coronary angiography indicated a persistent trend of improvement in both treatment groups when reexamined 6–24 hr after the second infusion and at hospital discharge. There was a greater reduction in plaque area in patients given prolonged rt-PA treatment (21).

IX. PATENCY RATE AND REGIONAL WALL MOTION AFTER 3 MONTHS

All patients who entered the rt-PA versus placebo trial (1) in one center were reexamined after approximately 3 months, using the same catheterization technique (22). The coronary and left ventricle angiograms were analyzed without knowledge of the treatment given at the acute stage of myocardial infarction. The angiographic criteria used by the local investigators for assessing the patency of the infarct-related vessel are those applied in the two collaborative trials (1,2). Regional wall motion of the infarct-related area was quantitated with digital subtraction angiography. The left ventricle cavity borders were outlined manually on the images at end diastole and end systole. Global ejection was calculated from the traced silhouettes according to the area-length method as described in detail elsewhere (22).

In the placebo group, the patency rates at the end of infusion and at 3 months' followup were 21 (three of 14 patients) and 58% (eight of 14 patients), respectively. Thus, late spontaneous thrombolysis occurred in five of 11 placebo patients (46%). This delayed reopening rate is less than the one reported by Rentrop et al. 2 weeks after acute myocardial infarction (23). The late reocclusion rate of 17% (two of 12 patients) in the rt-PA group is in the range reported after intracoronary or intravenous streptokinase (16,17). In both the placebo and the rt-PA groups, a nonsignificant improvement in global ejection fraction and a significant improvement in wall motion were found. These results are at variance with those obtained from radionuclide ventriculography (24). When the data of this small subgroup of patients of the collaborative trial are analyzed on the basis of patency, irrespective of treatment allocation, patients with an open infarct-related vessel in the acute phase and at 3-month followup showed a significant improvement in both global and regional left ventricle function, while patients with a persistent occlusion showed no change, as previously demonstrated by Sheehan et al. (25).

Antibodies against rt-PA were not detected in serum 2 weeks after rt-PA infusion (22). These results demonstrate the lack of antigenicity of rt-PA produced by a nonhuman mammalian cell line and indicate the possibility of repeated effective thrombolysis with this drug.

X. TWO EUROPEAN STUDIES IN PROGRESS OF LEFT VENTRICULAR FUNCTION

The data provided by studies on the early thrombolytic treatment in acute myocardial infarction are compatible with improved followup, although the number of patients studied in most centers is too small to warrant definitive conclusions (26,27). The largest trial to date, of 533 patients, demonstrated limitation of infarct size by 30% (HBDH release), preservation of left ventricular function (contrast and radionuclide angiography) and improved 1-year survival after intracoronary streptokinase (91% versus 84% in randomized controls) in patients admitted 4 hr after the onset of symptoms, although the number of nonfatal reinfarctions increased, in particular in patients with right coronary artery disease (28,29). It may be postulated that the beneficial effects of recanalization in acute myocardial infarction will be related to the speed and extent of recanalization and to the number of patent arteries after intervention. However, no data are yet available to define the cost-benefit relationship of the various interventions.

In order to determine whether patients with acute myocardial infarction benefit from early intravenous administration of rt-PA alone or from rt-PA immediately followed by percutaneous transluminal coronary angioplasty, two related clinical trials are being performed in Europe. The protocol of the first study investigates whether early intravenous administration of rt-PA reduces infarct size (estimated by serial myocardial enzyme release), preserves left ventricular function (measured by contrast angiography), and improves clinical state and long-term prognosis in comparison with placebo treatment.

Since several investigators believe that thrombolysis is only the first step toward effective myocardial reperfusion, which should be followed by immediate or early angioplasty (or bypass surgery), the protocol of the second trial explores whether further benefit can be obtained when mechanical perforation and angioplasty are performed in addition to intravenous administration of rt-PA.

Thus, the first protocol compares in a double-blind manner the relative value of conventional treatment in CCUs with infusion of placebo, with conventional treatment supplemented by intravenous administration of rt-PA. The second protocol compares conventional treatment supplemented by intravenous administration of rt-PA, with intravenous administration of rt-PA immediately followed by coronary angiography and coronary angioplasty. Each of the participating hospitals participates in either protocol I (rt-PA versus placebo) or protocol II (rt-PA versus rt-PA with additional PTCA). Randomization is balanced in each hospital, so that overall a quarter of the patients will receive placebo treatment, half of the patients intravenous rt-PA, and the remaining quarter will receive intravenous rt-PA followed by angiography and coronary angioplasty.

APPENDIX

Steering Committee of the European Cooperative Study Group for Recombinant Tissue-Type Plasminogen Activator:

> M. Verstraete (chairman)
> R. J. Lennane
> D. P. de Bono
> J. Lubsen
> D. Mathey
> W. Rutsch
> P. W. Serruys
> F. Van de Werf
> A. Vahanian
> R. von Essen

Advisory Board
> J. Hampton
> J. Jesdinsky
> D. G. Julian
> W. Schaper
> L. Wilhelmsen

Data Center
> J. Lubsen
> R. W. Brower
> A. E. R. Arnold
> B. Bos-Wolvers
> M. Bokslag
> Thorax Center Rotterdam

Angiography Evaluation Group
> D. P. de Bono (secretary)
> W. S. Hillis
> D. Reid
> C. Turnbull

Central Coagulation Laboratory
> D. Collen
> H. R. Lijnen

REFERENCES

1. Verstraete M, Bleifeld W, Brower RW, Charbonnier B, Collen D, de Bono DP, Dunning AJ, Lennane RJ, Lubsen J, Mathey DG, Michel PL, Raynaud Ph, Schofer J, Vahanian A, Vanhaecke J, Van de Kley GA, Van de Werf F, von Essen R: Double-blind, randomised trial of intravenous tissue-type plasminogen activator versus placebo in acute myocardial infarction. Lancet 2:965–969, 1985.

2. Verstraete M, Bernard R, Bory M, Brower RW, Collen D, de Bono DP, Erbel R, Huhmann W, Lennane RJ, Lubsen J, Mathey D, Meyer J, Michels HR, Rutsch W, Schartl M, Schmidt W, Uebis R, von Essen R: Randomised trial of intravenous recombinant tissue-type plasminogen activator versus intravenous streptokinase in acute myocardial infarction. Lancet 1:842–847, 1985.

3. Vermylen C, De Vreker RA, Verstraete M: A rapid enzymatic method for the assay of fibrinogen: the fibrin polymerization test (F.P.T.). Clin Chim Acta 8:418–424, 1963.

4. Rampling WF, Gaffney PJ: The sulphite precipitation method for fibrinogen measurement: its use on small samples in the presence of fibrinogen degradation products. Clin Chim Acta 67:43–52, 1976.

5. Merskey C, Lalezari P, Johnson AJ: A rapid, simple, sensitive method for measuring fibrinolytic split products in human serum. Proc Soc Exp Biol Med 131:871–878, 1969.

6. Rijken DC, Juhan-Vague I, De Cock F, Collen D: Measurement of human tissue-type plasminogen activator by a two-site immunoradiometric assay. J Lab Clin Med 101:274–294, 1983.

7. Collen D, Bounameaux H, De Cock F, Verstraete M: Analysis of coagulation and fibrinolysis during intravenous infusion of recombinant human tissue-type plasminogen activator (rt-PA) in patents with acute myocardial infarction. Circulation 73:511–517, 1986.

8. Rijken DC, Juhan-Vague I, Collen D: Complexes between tissue-type plasminogen activator and proteinase inhibitors in human plasma, identified with immunoradiometric assay. J Lab Clin Med 101:285–294, 1983.

9. Verstraete M, Su CAPF, Tanswell P, Feuerer W, Collen D: Pharmacokinetics and effects on fibrinolytic and coagulation parameters of two doses of recombinant tissue-type plasminogen activator in healthy volunteers. Thromb Haemost, August 1986, in press.

10. Verstraete M, Bounameaux H, De Cock F, Van de Werf F, Collen D: Pharmacokinetics and systemic fibrinogenolytic effects of recombinant human tissue-type plasminogen activator (rt-PA) in man. J Pharmacol Exp Ther 235:506–512, 1985.

11. Korninger C, Collen D: Studies on the specific fibrinolytic effect of human extrinsic tissue-type plasminogen activator in human blood and in various animal species in vitro. Thromb Haemost 46:561–565, 1981.

12. Fuchs HE, Berger H, Pizzo SV: Catabolism of human tissue-plasminogen activator in mice. Blood 65:539–544, 1985.

13. Bounameaux H, Stassen JM, Seghers C, Collen D: Influence of fibrin and liver blood flow on the turnover and the systemic fibrinogenolytic effects of recombinant human tissue-type plasminogen activator in rabbits. Blood 67:1493–1497, 1986.

14. Hoylaerts M, Rijken DC, Lijnen HR, Collen D: Kinetics of the activation of plasminogen by human tissue plasminogen activator. J Biol Chem 257:2912–2919, 1982.

15. Garabedian H, Gold HK, Leinbach RC, Yasuda T, Johns JA, Collen D: Coronary thrombolysis with recombinant human tissue-type plasminogen activator: dose dependent thrombolysis, pharmacokinetics, and hemostatic effects. Am Heart J, in press.

16. Spann JF, Sherry S: Coronary thrombolysis for evolving myocardial infarction. Drugs 28:465–483, 1984.

17. Erbel R, Pop T, Meinerts T, Kasper W, Schreiner G, Henkel B, Henrichs KJ, Pfeiffer C, Rupprecht HJ, Meyer J: Combined medical and mechanical recanalization in acute myocardial infarction. Cathet Cardiovasc Diagn 11:361–377, 1985.

18. Williams DO, Borer J, Braunwald E, Chesebro JH, Cohen LS, Dalen J, Dodge HT, Francis CK, Knatterud G, Ludbrook P, Markis JE, Mueller H, Desvigne-Nickens P, Passamani ER, Powers ER, Rao AK, Roberts R, Ross A, Ryan TJ, Sobel BE, Winniford M, Zaret B, et al: Intravenous recombinant tissue-type plasminogen activator in patients with acute myocardial infarction: a report from the NHLBI thrombolysis in myocardial infarction trial. Circulation 73:338–346, 1986.

19. Gold HK, Leinbach RC, Garabedian HD, Yasuda T, Johns JA, Grossbard EB, Palacios I, Collen D: Acute coronary reocclusion after thrombolysis with recombinant human tissue-type plasminogen activator: prevention by a maintenance infusion. Circulation 73:347–352, 1986.

20. Verstraete M, Arnold AER, Brower RW, Collen D, de Bono DP, de Zwaan C, Erbel R, Hillis WS, Lennane RJ, Lubsen J, Mathey D, Reid DS, Rutsch W, Schartl M, Serruys PW, Simoons ML, Uebis R, Vahanian A, Verheugt FWA, von Essen R: Acute coronary thrombolysis with recombinant human tissue-type plasminogen activator. Initial patency and influence of maintained infusion on occlusion rate. Lancet, submitted, 1986.

21. Serruys PW, Arnold AER, de Bono DP, Bokslag M, Lubsen J, Reiber JHC, Rutsch W, Uebis R, Vahanian A, Verstraete M: Effect of continued rt-PA administration on the residual stenosis after initially successful recanalization in acute myocardial infarction—a quantitative coronary angiography study of a randomised trial, submitted.

22. Jang IK, Vanhaecke J, De Geest H, Verstraete M, Collen D, Van de Werf F: Coronary thrombolysis with recombinant tissue-type plasminogen activator (rt-PA): patency rate and regional wall motion after 3 months. J Am Coll Cardiol, in press.

23. Rentrop KP, Feit F, Blanke H, Stecy P, Schneider R, Rey M, Horowitz S, Goldman M, Karsch K, Meilman H, Cohen M, Siegel S, Sanger J, Slater J, Gorlin R, Fox A, Fagerstrom R, Calhoun WF: Effects of intracoronary streptokinase and intracoronary nitroglycerin infusion on coronary angiographic patterns and mortality in patients with acute myocardial infarction. N Engl J Med 311:1457–1463, 1984.

24. Khaja F, Walton JA, Brymer JF, Lo E, Osterberger L, O'Neill WW, Colfer HT, Weiss R, Lee T, Kurian T, Goldberg D, Pitt B, Goldstein S: Intracoronary fibrinolytic therapy in acute myocardial infarction. Report of a prospective randomized trial. N Engl J Med 308:1305–1311, 1983.

25. Sheehan FH, Mathey DG, Schofer J, Kreber HJ, Dodge HT: Effect of interventions in salvaging left ventricular function in acute myocardial infarction: a study of intracoronary streptokinase. Am J Cardiol 52:431–438, 1983.

26. Yusuf S, Collins R, Peto R, Furberg C, Stampfer MJ, Goldhaber SZ, Hennekens CH: Intravenous and intracoronary fibrinolytic therapy in acute myocardial infarction: Overview of results on mortality, reinfarction and side-effects from 33 randomized controlled trials. Eur Heart J 6:556–585, 1985.

27. Verstraete M: Intravenous administration of a thrombolytic agent is the only realistic therapeutic approach in evolving myocardial infarction. Eur Heart J 6:586–593, 1985.

28. Simoons PW, Van den Brand M, Zwaan C, Verheugt FWA, Serruys PW, Bär F, Res J, Krauss XH, Vermeer F, Lubsen J: Improved survival after early thrombolysis in acute myocardial infarction. A randomized trial conducted by the Interuniversity Cardiology Institute in The Netherlands. Lancet 2:578–582, 1985.

29. Simoons ML, Serruys PW, Van den Brand M, Res J, Verheugt FWA, Krauss XH, Rimme WJ, Bär F, de Zwaan C, van der Laarse A, Vermeer F, Lubsen J: Early thrombolysis in acute myocardial infarction: limitation of infarct size and improved survival. J Am Coll Cardiol 7:717–728, 1986.

12

Thrombolytic Therapy in Japan: Urokinase Infusion for Acute Myocardial Infarction

Hirofumi Kambara and Chuichi Kawai
Kyoto University
Kyoto, Japan

I. INTRODUCTION

Since 1979, when Rentrop et al. (1) introduced intracoronary infusion of streptokinase, there have been striking changes in the early management of acute myocardial infarction. In the past, therapies for acute myocardial infarction were directed toward the complications of infarction. The aims of the new thrombolytic therapy are the restoration of coronary artery blood flow, reduction of infarct size, preservation of left ventricular function, and reduction of mortality.

Horie et al. (2) evaluated 108 autopsied cases by examining serial sections of the coronary arteries and concluded that the rupture of atheroma and subsequent thrombosis were the main causes of infarction. DeWood et al. (3) documented the presence of coronary thrombosis in the majority of patients with acute transmural myocardial infarction, 90% within 4 hr after the onset of chest pain and 60% in 24 hr. Therefore, intracoronary thrombolysis should be feasible for the majority of patients with acute myocardial infarction. In Japan, intracoronary thrombolytic therapy employing urokinase has been used since 1981, and the results will be summarized in this chapter.

II. JAPANESE MULTICENTER OPEN TRIAL OF INTRACORONARY UROKINASE ADMINISTRATION IN ACUTE MYOCARDIAL INFARCTION

A Japanese multicenter study of intracoronary urokinase administration was started in 1982, and the results were reported in 1984 by Kawai (4) and in 1985 by Kambara et al. (5). Thirty cardiovascular centers participated in this study and a total of 514 cases were registered. Myocardial infarction was defined by chest pain of 30 min or more in duration that could not be relieved by nitrates, ST elevation of more than 2 mm in more than one lead, and subsequent elevation of cardiac enzymes. Coronary angiography could be adequately evaluated in 500 cases, which included 405 men and 95 women; the patients' ages ranged from 27 to 86 years (average 59). Two hundred and eighty-eight had anterior, 191 had inferior, and 21 had posterolateral infarction. The average time between the onset of chest pain and coronary angiography was 5 hr, range 0.5 to 81 hr. Urokinase was administered by bolus or continuous injection, either intracoronary or into the sinus of Valsalva. Coronary angiography demonstrated that these treatments were effective in 66.8% of the cases and were far more effective than the use of nitrates alone (9.3%).

Usually, 240,000 units of urokinase is infused slowly every 10 min, with the total dose up to 960,000 units. The smaller the dose, the worse the results, and a total dose of more than 480,000 units is necessary to achieve a good success rate (Table 1). Continuous infusion into the sinus of Valsalva was also effective in 63% of the cases.

Recanalization rates at various intervals after the onset of chest pain indicated that the successful recanalization occurred in 76.7% of the cases in which the urokinase infusion was started within 2 hr after the onset of pain; this recanalization rate is better than that found in the rest of the cases (64.2%,

Table 1   Efficacy of Coronary Thrombolysis with Intracoronary Urokinase Administration

Dose of urokinase ($\times$1000 IU)	$\geq$240	241–480	481–720	721–960	$\geq$961
No. of cases	146	142	148	40	24
Successful cases	104	108	93	20	9
Cumulative successful cases (%)	104/500 (20.8)	212/500 (42.4)	305/500 (61)	325/500 (65)	334/500 (66.8)

$p < 0.05$). However, recanalization did occur even in cases where the therapy was started from 6 to 81 hr after the onset of pain. Thus, the ability to achieve successful thrombolysis was somewhat influenced by the time between the onset of chest pain and coronary arteriography.

Reperfusion occurred in 68.0% of the left anterior descending coronary artery occlusions, 67.6% of the right coronary artery occlusions, and 53.8% in the left circumflex artery occlusions. Proximal occlusions of the infarct vessels were more easily recanalized than mid- or distal coronary occlusions (75.8%, 66.4%, and 56.3%, respectively).

The adverse effects directly related to the procedure are listed in Table 2. The number of arrhythmias was greater in the patients with successful thrombolysis as compared to those in whom the procedure was unsuccessful, but the clinical responses to antiarrhythmic medications were generally better in the former than in the latter. Serious hemorrhage requiring blood transfusion was rare, and no death directly related to this treatment was reported.

The electrocardiographic changes after coronary thrombolysis revealed significant improvement in the ST changes in the successful cases [144/334 (43.1%) in the successful cases versus 33/166 (19.9%) in unsuccessful cases; $p < 0.001$]. There was an increased number of leads with abnormal Q waves in the successful cases (129/334, 55.6%) than among the unsuccessful cases (42/166, 25.3%; $p < 0.05$).

The hospital deaths were less frequent in patients with successful throm-

Table 2   Adverse Effects of Intracoronary Administration of Urokinase

	Thrombolysis	
Adverse effects	Successful (334 cases)	Unsuccessful (166 cases)
Arrhythmia	111 (33.2%)	18 (10.8%)
Chest pain with ST elevation	2 (0.6%)	2 (1.2%)
Cardiogenic shock	1 (0.3%)	0
Respiratory arrest	2 (0.6%)	1 (0.6%)
Drug-induced hemorrhage	1 (0.3%)	1 (1.2%)
Others	5 (1.5%)	3 (1.8%)
Total	122 (36.5%)	25 (15.1%)

bolysis than in those with unsuccessful thrombolysis (6.3 versus 13.3%). The reinfarction rates during hospitalization were similar in the two groups (2.1% in the successful group and 2.4% in the unsuccessful group).

III. FOLLOWUP STUDY AFTER INTRACORONARY THROMBOLYSIS IN ACUTE MYOCARDIAL INFARCTION

Twelve cardiovascular centers participated in this study and 315 cases were registered. Twenty-four patients who underwent major therapeutic procedures such as acute coronary bypass procedures, angioplasty, and/or intraaortic balloon pumping were excluded, and 291 cases were analyzed. The study population consisted of 246 male and 45 female patients, with an average age of 59.1 ± 9.1 (SD) years. Two hundred and thirty-six patients had total occlusions prior to thrombolysis and 55 patients had subtotal occlusions. Coronary thrombolysis with intracoronary urokinase administration was effective in 107 cases (63.2%).

The followup periods ranged from 7 to 243 weeks, with an average of 95 weeks. Left heart catheterization was performed in 235 cases, approximately 1 month after the thrombolytic procedure. Twenty patients died before the repeat catheterization.

The left ventricular ejection fraction was 51.1 ± 13.9% in the successful thrombolysis group and 47.2 ± 13.2% in the unsuccessful group, without a statistical difference between the two. However, in the patients admitted within 3 hr after the onset of pain, the successful thrombolysis group demonstrated a better ejection fraction (53.3 ± 12.5%) than the unsuccessful group (43.9 ± 15.0%; p < 0.05). There were no significant differences in other hemodynamic parameters such as the cardiac index or the left ventricular end-

Table 3   Recanalization Time and Number of Cardiac Deaths

Recanalization time after onset of chest pain	No. of cases	Cardiac deaths (%)
Within 3 hr	78	4 (5.1)
Within 6 hr	146	11 (7.5)
After 6 hr and unsuccessful cases[a]	132	14 (10.6)

[a]15 cases lost to followup.

Table 4   Residual Coronary Stenosis and Cardiac Deaths

Residual stenosis after thrombolysis	No. of cases	Cardiac deaths (%)
≤75%	23	0 (0)
76–90%	85	6 (7.1)
91–99%	88	9 (10.2)
100%	82	10 (12.2)
Total	278	25 (9)

diastolic pressure, but earlier recanalization tended to reduce cardiac mortality (Table 3). The absence of a statistical difference in the hemodynamic parameters is due partly to the inhomogeneity of the groups of patients studied with respect to collaterals, degree of recanalization, persistence of recanalization, and other clinical parameters. There was some evidence that the more severe the residual stenosis after coronary thrombolysis in the acute phase, the higher the mortality (Table 4).

Thus, early recanalization is beneficial and residual stenosis plays an important role in the long-term prognosis.

IV. RANDOMIZED DOUBLE-BLIND TRIAL OF INTRACORONARY UROKINASE INFUSION

To assess the efficacy of intracoronary urokinase administration in patients with acute myocardial infarction, a double-blind study with urokinase and placebo was undertaken in 64 hospitals between 1984 and 1985 (6). The selection criteria included: 1) admission within 6 hr after the onset of chest pain and 2) total occlusion of the infarct-related artery on coronary arteriography after the administration of intracoronary nitrates. Two hundred and ten patients met the criteria; 107 patients were randomized to receive intracoronary urokinase and 103 to receive placebo. After a bolus injection of heparin 5000 U intravenously, one vial of either urokinase 120,000 IU or placebo was administered every 5 min, up to eight vials. After each intracoronary administration of two vials, coronary arteriography was repeated to evaluate the patency of the arteries.

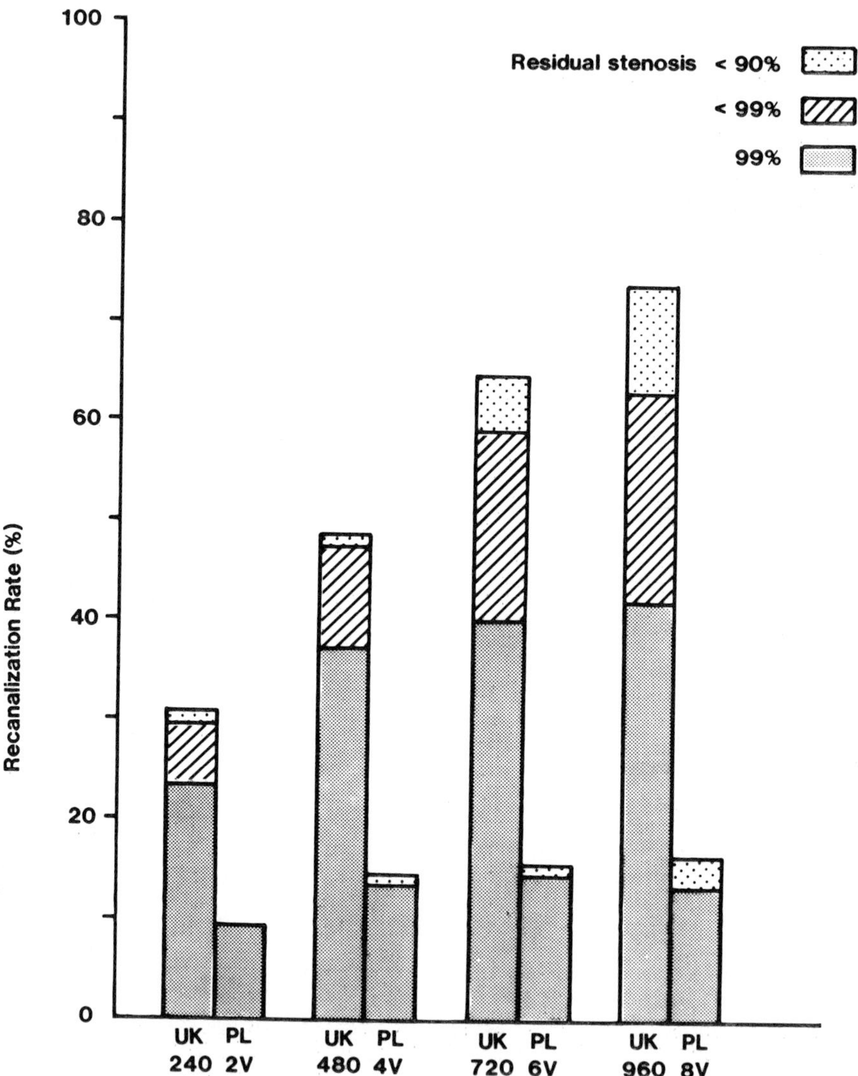

Figure 1   Relationship between the administration dosage of urokinase (UK) and the recanalization rate. Dosage UK: ×1000 IU. Dosage placebo (PL): vials.

Reopening of the infarct-related arteries was achieved in 79 of 107 cases (73.8%) in the urokinase group and 17 of 103 cases (16.5%) in the placebo group (p < 0.01). Figure 1 demonstrates the recanalization rates as a function of the dosage of urokinase. The recanalization rate varied directly with the dose, up to 960,000 IU in the urokinase group.

The success rate for the alleviation of chest pain at the end of the study was higher in the urokinase group (47.6%) than in the placebo group (19.8%). Hemodynamically, the cardiac index showed no significant change in either group, but the left ventricular end-diastolic pressure was slightly reduced from 20.7 ± 8.8 mm Hg at the beginning of the study to 20.0 ± 7.1 mm Hg at the end of the study in the urokinase group, and slightly increased from 17.3 ± 7.0 to 21.8 ± 6.9 mm Hg in the placebo group, with a significant difference between the two groups (Table 5).

One hundred and sixty-five of the 210 patients registered had repeat coronary arteriography approximately 1 month postinfarction and 134 cases (81.2%) showed patent coronary arteries. Because additional thrombolytic or angioplastic procedures after the double-blind study were allowed as part of the recanalization procedure, statistical analysis between the urokinase and placebo groups was not appropriate. However, the patients with persistent recanalization had better ejection fractions (55.7 ± 12.9%) than did those with occluded coronary arteries (47.6 ± 10.7%; p < 0.05). Sixteen patients (7.6%) died during the initial month postinfarction; all deaths were of cardiac etiology. Patients with early recanalization (less than 4 hr after the onset of

Table 5   Hemodynamic Changes During the Study Periods

Hemodynamic parameters	Urokinase group		Placebo group	
Cardiac index (L/min/m²)	2.92 ± 0.99	→ 3.12 ± 0.98	2.91 ± 0.87	→ 3.14 ± 1.10
		NS		
Left ventricular end-diastolic pressure (mm Hg)	20.7 ± 8.8	→ 20.0 ± 7.1	17.3 ± 7.0	→ 21.8 ± 6.9
		p < 0.05		

pain) had a lower 1-month mortality rate (3.5%) than did the patients with total coronary occlusion lasting for more than 4 hr (16.2%; p < 0.05).

Thus, this double-blind study showed that early administration of urokinase could reestablish coronary flow in a high proportion of patients and that early thrombolysis with persistent recanalization appeared to lead to a significantly better outcome.

V. CORONARY THROMBOLYSIS WITH INTRAVENOUS ADMINISTRATION OF UROKINASE

In 1983 and 1984, the efficacy of intravenous administration of a large amount of urokinase was investigated in a double-blind fashion in patients with acute myocardial infarction by Hirosawa, Kawai, and colleagues.

Consecutive patients with acute transmural myocardial infarction were studied in 22 cardiovascular centers. All patients had had the onset of chest pain 6 hr or less before admission and had persistent pain and ST-segment elevation despite the administration of nitrates. The patients were blindly assigned to a low-dose urokinase (480,000 IU) group or a high-dose (980,000 IU) group. Fifty-eight patients were analyzed, including 26 in the low-dose group (age range 42 to 74 years; mean 56.9 years) and 32 in the high-dose group (age range 41 to 80 years; mean 57.7 years). The mean duration between the onset of chest pain and hospitalization was 211 min in the low-dose group and 236 min in the high-dose group.

Urokinase was infused intravenously over 30 min when total occlusion was noted angiographically despite the administration of nitrates. Coronary arteriography was repeated 30 min after completion of the urokinase infusion, and recanalization was found in 13.6% of the low-dose group and in 50.0% of the high-dose group, with a significant difference between the two groups. Residual coronary stenosis was also more severe in the low-dose group (Table 6).

In 1985, additional intravenous urokinase studies were undertaken in nine hospitals to assess the patency rate after a very high dose of urokinase. Twenty-three cases with an administration dose of 1,200,000 IU were studied by coronary arteriography. Successful recanalization occurred in 13 cases (56.5%). Three (13.0%) developed hemorrhagic complications that required blood transfusion. The other 17 cases with or without coronary arteriography were given 1,400,000–1,920,000 IU of urokinase, and 13 cases (76.5%) showed evidence of recanalization. However, this large dose induced an unacceptably high frequency of hemorrhagic complications (more than 40%). Therefore, the appropriate dosage of intravenous urokinase for coronary thrombolysis is considered to be between 960,000 and 1,200,000 IU.

Table 6   Intravenous Urokinase Infusion and Recanalization Rate

Dose (IU)	Recanalization rate (%)	Residual stenosis (% of cases)		
		99%	98–90%	<90%
480,000	13.6	66.7	33.3	0
960,000	50.0	38.5	53.8	7.7

VI. CLINICAL BENEFITS

Contraction band necrosis is a well-documented pathological phenomenon after reperfusion, but its clinical significance is unclear. Reperfusion hemorrhage has also been described after long periods of ischemia. This hemorrhage is considered to be due to the combined effects of reperfusion and large doses of urokinase. However, it is unlikely that hemorrhage expands the infarct area or exacerbates the clinical condition (7).

Some data suggest that coronary artery reperfusion exerts a beneficial effect in acute transmural infarction by reducing infarct size (8–10), improving left ventricular function (10–13), and reducing mortality (5, 14–16). These effects greatly depend on the time lag between the onset of chest pain and reperfusion. We assessed 30 patients with a first anterior myocardial infarction who had undergone intracoronary thrombolysis (17). The patients were divided into three groups on the basis of the occlusion time of the left anterior descending coronary artery: 4 hr or less (11 patients), 4–10 hr (11 patients), and 10 hr or more (eight patients). Serial measurements of serum creatine kinase-MB were carried out in the acute phase. Four weeks after the thrombolysis, pathological Q waves on 34-lead precordial mapping were scored electrocardiographically, myocardial infarct volume was estimated by ^{201}Tl myocardial emission computed tomography, and left ventricular function was evaluated by contrast ventriculography. The results indicated that infarct size increased and left ventricular function deteriorated with increasing duration of occlusion of the left anterior descending coronary artery, and that not only early ($\leq$4 hr) but also later (4–10 hr) reperfusion was beneficial in preventing the enlargement of the infarction and the deterioration of left ventricular function in patients with anterior infarctions.

Further extension of the study in 106 cases demonstrated that the patients who had the greatest benefit from reperfusion were those at high risk with left anterior descending coronary artery thrombosis (Table 7). In this

Table 7   Occlusion Periods of Each Coronary Artery and Infarct Size

Occlusion periods	ΣCK-MB (IU)	^{201}Tl defect score	LVEF (%)
Left anterior descending artery (58 cases)			
$\leq$4 hr	170 ± 119[a]	13 ± 6[a]	55 ± 8[a]
4–10 hr	332 ± 101	40 ± 9[b]	52 ± 10[b]
$\geq$10 hr or unsuccessful thrombolysis	587 ± 197	55 ± 17	40 ± 14
Right coronary artery (30 cases)			
$\leq$4 hr	134 ± 85[b]	12 ± 8[a]	49 ± 10
4–10 hr	209 ± 110	24 ± 8	48 ± 14
$\geq$10 hr or unsuccessful thrombolysis	263 ± 78	31 ± 11	46 ± 12
Left circumflex artery (18 cases)			
$\leq$4 hr	155 ± 100	15 ± 9[b]	60 ± 8
4–10 hr	201 ± 65	24 ± 10	58 ± 10
$\geq$10 hr or unsuccessful thrombolysis	203 ± 110	26 ± 11	54 ± 12

Comparison with $\geq$10 hr or unsuccessful thrombolysis cases.
[a]$p < 0.01$.
[b]$p < 0.05$.

study, a ^{201}Tl defect score was obtained by adding the defect scores, graded from 0 to 3 in each segment. Myocardial tomographic images were divided into 52 segments. In patients with successful thrombolysis in the left anterior descending coronary artery, early ($\leq$4 hr) and even later (4–10 hr) recanalization exerted beneficial effects, but only early recanalization appeared to have some benefits in patients who had thrombolysis in the right coronary and left circumflex arteries. These findings are concordant with those of Kennedy et al. (16).

The improvement in myocardial function postinfarction is also influenced by the number of collaterals to the infarct-related arteries (18) and by the degree of stenosis in the arteries that supply the collaterals (19).

VII. CURRENT INVESTIGATIONS

Combined treatments with urokinase and percutaneous transluminal coronary angioplasty (PTCA) are actively under investigation in many Japanese cardiovascular centers. Successful PTCA with sustained patency of the infarct-related coronary artery may have a beneficial effect in salvaging the jeopardized myocardium (20). Our previous data also suggest that a high degree of residual narrowing after thrombolysis has serious potential consequences (Table 4). PTCA could be performed safely after urokinase therapy in patients with acute myocardial infarction. The effect of PTCA may be complementary and desirable by virtue of its potential to provide more complete revascularization of the infarct zone, but there is an increased hazard of inducing reocclusion in the acute phase compared with PTCA performed in the chronic phase.

A major theoretical advantage of tissue-type plasminogen activator (t-PA) compared to first-generation lytic agents relates to its fibrin selectivity. The ability of t-PA to dissolve coronary thrombus has been approximately 75%, which compares favorably to the 50 to 55% efficacy rate of intravenous streptokinase or urokinase. However, a very high dose of t-PA may induce hemorrhage. Furthermore, the short time span of fibrinolysis with t-PA may result in reocclusion of the coronary arteries involved.

Other second-generation lytic agents include pro-urokinase and acylated streptokinase-plasminogen activator. Pro-urokinase has been investigated in more than 60 patients and the efficacy of intracoronary administration is well documented. Controlled trials of the intravenous use of this agent are currently under way.

VIII. SUMMARY

Intracoronary urokinase administration is a safe and effective means of coronary thrombolysis. Reperfusion occurred in 68% of the left anterior descending coronary artery occlusions, 67.6% of the right coronary artery occlusions, and 53.8% of the left circumflex artery occlusions. Overall, in Japan, successful thrombolysis with intracoronary urokinase was achieved in 66.8% of 500 patients with acute myocardial infarction. This efficacy was firmly established in our randomized study of urokinase versus placebo with recanalization rates of 73.8% versus 16.5%, respectively. Early recanalization was beneficial, but the degree of residual stenosis was an important factor in the long-term prognosis.

REFERENCES

1. Rentrop KP, Blanke H, Karsch KR, Kreuzer H: Initial experience with transluminal recanalization of the recently occluded infarct-related coronary artery in acute myocardial infarction: comparison with conventionally treated patients. Clin Cardiol 2:92–105, 1979.

2. Horie T, Sekiguchi M, Hirosawa K: Coronary thrombosis in pathogenesis of acute myocardial infarction: histopathological study of coronary arteries in 108 necropsied cases using serial section. Br Heart J 40:153–161, 1978.

3. DeWood MA, Spores J, Notske R, Mouser LT, Burroughs R, Golden MS, Lang HT: Prevalence of total coronary occlusion during the early hours of transmural myocardial infarction. N Engl J Med 303:897–902, 1980.

4. Kawai C: New horizons in cardiology. Int J Cardiol 6:569–579, 1984.

5. Kambara H, Kawai C, Kammatsuse K, Sato H, Nobuyoshi M, Chino M, Miwa H, Uchida Y, Kodama K, Mitsudo K, Hayashi T, Kajiwara N, Sekiguchi M, Yasue H: Coronary thrombolysis with urokinase infusion in acute myocardial infarction: multicenter study in Japan. Cathet Cardiovasc Diagn 11:349–360, 1985.

6. Kambara H, Kammatsuse K, Nobuyoshi M, Kodama K, Sato H, Sasayama S, Kajiwara N, Nakajima M, Kawai C: Randomized double-blind trial of intracoronary urokinase for acute myocardial infarction: multicenter study. Jpn Circ J 51, 1987 (in press).

7. Fujiwara H, Onodera T, Tanaka M, Fujiwara T, Wu Der-J, Kawai C: A clinicopathologic study of patients with hemorrhagic myocardial infarction treated with selective coronary thrombolysis with urokinase. Circulation 73:749–757, 1986.

8. Renduto LA, Freund GC, Gaeta JM, Smalling RW, Lewis B, Gould KL: Coronary artery reperfusion in acute myocardial infarction: beneficial effects of intracoronary streptokinase of left ventricular salvage and performance. Am Heart J 102:1168–1177, 1981.

9. Schwarz F, Schuler G, Katus H, Hofmann M, Manthey J, Tillmanns H, Mehmel HC, Kubler W: Intracoronary thrombolysis in acute myocardial infarction: duration of ischemia as a major determinant of late results after recanalization. Am J Cardiol 50:933–937, 1982.

10. Tamaki S, Murakami T, Kadota K, Kambara H, Yui Y, Nakajima H, Suzuki Y, Nohara R, Kawai C, Tamaki M, Mukai T, Torizuka K: Effects of coronary artery reperfusion on relation between creatine kinase-MB release and infarct size estimated by myocardial emission tomography with thallium-201 in man. J Am Coll Cardiol 2:1031–1033, 1983.

11. Khaja F, Walton JA, Brymer JF, Lo E, Osterberger L, O'Neill WW, Colfer HT, Weiss R, Lee T, Kurian T, Goldberg AD, Pitt B, Goldstein S: Intracoronary fibrinolytic therapy in acute myocardial infarction: report of a prospective randomized trial. N Engl J Med 308:1305–1311, 1983.

12. Anderson JL, Marshall HW, Bray BE, Lutz JR, Frederick PR, Yanowitz FG, Datz FL, Klausner SC, Hagan AD: A randomized trial of intracoronary streptokinase in the treatment of acute myocardial infarction. N Engl J Med 308: 1312–1318, 1983.

13. Kennedy JW, Ritchie JL, Davies K, Fritz JK: Western Washington randomized trial of intracoronary streptokinase in acute myocardial infarction. N Engl J Med 309:1477–1482, 1983.

14. Timmis GC, Gangadharan V, Hauser AM, Ramos RG, Westveer DG, Gordon S: Intracoronary streptokinase in clinical practice. Am Heart J 104:925–938, 1982.

15. Weinstein J: The international registry to support approval of intracoronary streptokinase thrombolysis in the treatment of acute myocardial infarction. Circulation 68(suppl I):61–66, 1983.

16. Kennedy JW, Gensini GG, Timmis GC, Maynard C: Acute myocardial infarction treated with intracoronary streptokinase: a report of the Society for Cardiac Angiography. Am J Cardiol 55:871–877, 1985.

17. Murakami T, Kambara H, Kadota K, Tamaki S, Nakamura Y, Kishimoto C, Nohara R, Hattori R, Takatsu Y, Kawai C: Effects of intracoronary thrombolysis on infarct size and left ventricular function in patients with anterior myocardial infarction: enzymatic, electrocardiographic, radionuclide and hemodynamic evaluations. Jpn Circ J 49:605–615, 1985.

18. Saito Y, Yasuno M, Ishida M, Suzuki K, Matoba Y, Emura M, Takahashi M: Importance of coronary collaterals for restoration of left ventricular function after intracoronary thrombolysis. Am J Cardiol 55:1259–1263, 1985.

19. Nohara R, Kambara H, Murakami T, Kadota K, Tamaki S, Kawai C: Collateral function in early acute myocardial infarction. Am J Cardiol 52:955–959, 1983.

20. Yasuno M, Saito Y, Ishida M, Suzuki K, Endo S, Takahashi M: Effects of percutaneous transluminal coronary angioplasty: intracoronary thrombolysis with urokinase in acute myocardial infarction. Am J Cardiol 53:1217–1220, 1984.

Index

About the Editors

Burton E. Sobel is the Tobias and Hortense Lewin Distinguished Professor in Cardiovascular Disease at the Washington University School of Medicine in St. Louis, Missouri, where he has taught since 1973. He serves as Director of the Cardiovascular Division at the Washington University School of Medicine as well as at the Barnes and Wohl Hospitals in St. Louis, and he is Adjunct Professor of Chemistry at Washington University. The author or coauthor of over 420 articles and book chapters, he has lectured at universities and conferences throughout the world. He has served as Editor of the journals *Circulation* and *Clinical Cardiology*, and as an editorial board member of, among many others, the *Journal of Clinical Investigation, Annals of Internal Medicine, Circulation Research*, and *American Journal of Physiology: Heart and Circulatory Physiology*. He is a Fellow of The Royal Society of Medicine in the U.K., American College of Cardiology (which he served as Governor), and the American College of Physicians, and he is a member of numerous societies, including the American Society for Clinical Investigation, American Physiological Society, Society for Experimental Biology and Medicine, and Association of

University Cardiologists. Dr. Sobel received the A.B. degree (1958) from Cornell University and M.D. degree (1962) magna cum laude from Harvard Medical School.

Désiré Collen is Professor in the Faculty of Medicine at the University of Leuven in Belgium, where he serves in addition as Associate Head of Clinic at the University Hospitals. He is also Professor of Biochemistry and Medicine at the University of Vermont's College of Medicine and Visiting Professor at the Free University of Brussels in Belgium. His research focuses on the molecular biology and pathophysiology of hemostasis and thrombosis as well as the development of new thrombolytic and antithrombotic agents. A member of the Royal Academy of Medicine of Belgium, he has been awarded numerous honors for his work, including the Servier Prize for Research in Fibrinolysis (1978), A. Faes Prize (1981), Francqui Prize (1984), and the Louis Jeantet Prize for Medicine (1986). Since 1974 a higher associate in the Faculty of Medicine, Dr. Collen received the M.D. (1968), M.S. (1969; medical sciences), and Ph.D. (1974; chemistry) degrees from the Catholic University of Louvain.

Elliott B. Grossbard is Director of Clinical Research at Genentech, Inc., in South San Francisco, California. Previously he taught clinical medicine at Stanford University and Cornell University Medical Center, served as senior research physician at Hoffman-La Roche in Nutley, New Jersey, and was assistant director of the marrow transplant unit at Memorial Sloan-Kettering Cancer Center in New York City. The author or coauthor of 44 journal articles, book chapters, and abstracts, he is a member of the American Society of Hematology and American Heart Association. Dr. Grossbard received the B.A. degree (1969) from Columbia College, M.D. degree (1973) from Columbia University's College of Physicians and Surgeons, and M.S.L. degree (1981) from Yale University School of Law.